NEARLY 50 MILLION AMERICANS HAVE SOME FORM OF ARTHRITIS. IT IS THE COUNTRY'S NUMBER ONE CRIPPLING DISEASE. BUT, WITH TODAY'S SOPHISTICATED TREATMENTS, THE GREAT MAJORITY OF ITS VICTIMS CAN LEAD COMFORTABLE, ACTIVE LIVES.

The Pill Book of Arthritis, written especially for the consumer, tells you everything you need to know about the medications doctors prescribe for the treatment of the many forms of this disease. Here is the information right at your fingertips, including cautions and warnings, side effects, adverse reactions, usual dosage levels, and the potential for overdose. PLUS the causes of arthritis, the myths and realities of arthritis treatment, and how to live well with arthritis.

THE PILL BOOK OF ARTHRITIS

BERT STERN

Producer

LAWRENCE D. CHILNICK

Editor-in-Chief

TEXT BY
Vivienne Sernaqué

MEDICAL CONSULTANT
Israeli A. Jaffe, M.D.
Professor of Clinical Medicine,
College of Physicians and Surgeons,
Columbia University

ADDITIONAL TEXT/PRODUCTION
Daniel Montopoli

BANTAM BOOKS
TORONTO • NEW YORK • LONDON • SYDNEY • AUCKLAND

*Special acknowledgment to Tom Holdorf
for photography assistance.*

**Special thanks to Jeff Packer
and Dave Phillips, Carlyle Chemists,
New York City.**

THE PILL BOOK OF ARTHRITIS

A Bantam Book / March 1985

ISBN 0-553-24626-7

Published simultaneously in the United States and Canada

*Bantam Books are published by Bantam Books, Inc. Its
trademark, consisting of the words "Bantam Books" and the
portrayal of a rooster, is Registered in U.S. Patent and Trademark Office and in other countries. Marca Registrada. Bantam Books, Inc., 666 Fifth Avenue, New York, New York
10103.*

PRINTED IN THE UNITED STATES OF AMERICA

O   0 9 8 7 6 5 4 3 2 1   I

Contents

HOW TO USE THIS BOOK

The Pill Book of Arthritis is divided into three main sections:

1. Information about the many aspects of arthritis, including details about the nature of the disease, treatments both medical and nontraditional, and facts you should know about living with arthritis.

2. Easy-to-read profiles of the drugs most often prescribed to treat arthritis.

3. In addition, the book contains a section of life-sized pictures of the arthritis drugs most commonly prescribed in the United States.

The Pill Book of Arthritis's photo system for checking medications is designed to help you quickly identify the drug you're about to take. Included are the most popular brand-name drugs, and many of the drugs most frequently prescribed by generic name. Although several dosage levels may be included, other dosage levels may be omitted because they are prescribed less often.

The drugs are organized alphabetically and have

been reproduced as faithfully as possible. While every effort has been made to depict the drugs accurately, certain variations in size and color must be expected as a result of the photographic and printing processes. Therefore, you should never rely solely on the photographic image to identify any pill, but should check with your doctor or pharmacist if you have any questions whatsoever about the identification.

Most, but not all, of the drugs in the color section can be matched with your arthritis medication by matching your pill with the following on each photo:

- The imprinted company logo (i.e., "Lilly," "Roche")
- The product strength (i.e., "250 mg.," "10 mg.")
- The product code number, which may be imprinted on the pill

Because many generic drugs look the same as their brand-name counterparts, some manufacturers have started printing the product name on each pill.

To find out more about the drug shown, check the descriptive text on the pages referred to in the photo caption. The pill profiles provide complete descriptions of the most often prescribed generic and brand-name arthritis drugs. The descriptions give you detailed information about your prescriptions. The easy-to-read profiles are listed alphabetically by their generic names (except when the product profiled is a combination of two or more generic drugs; in which case, the popular brand names for these combinations are profiled in alphabetical order).

The drug profiles contain the following information:

Generic Name: The generic name is the drug's common name, or chemical name, as approved by the Food and Drug Administration (FDA).

Brand Name(s): The brand name is the name given by a particular drug company to identify its product. For example, Tylenol is a brand name for the generic drug acetaminophen. When particular drugs are also sold under their generic names, that information is included here.

Type of Drug: How the individual drug is classified, which may indicate its relation to other drugs. For example, Indocin, classed as a nonsteroidal anti-inflammatory drug (NSAID), is closely related to other NSAIDs such as Motrin, Ponstel, and Clinoril. Additional important information about these drug types is provided at the beginning of section II.

Prescribed for: The condition for which a drug is most often prescribed.

Cautions and Warnings: Any drug can be harmful if you are sensitive to any of its actions. The information provided here alerts you to possible allergic reactions, and to certain personal physical conditions, such as pregnancy and diabetes, which should be taken into consideration if the drug is prescribed for you.

Possible Side Effects: These are the more-common side effects to be expected from the drug.

Possible Adverse Effects: More-uncommon effects of a pill that may be cause for concern. If you are not sure whether you are experiencing an adverse reaction, ALWAYS CALL YOUR DOCTOR.

Drug Interactions: This section tells you which other drugs should be avoided when taking the arthritis pills. Drug interactions with other pills, alcohol, food, or other substances can cause death.

Interactions are more common than overdoses. It is very important to be careful when drinking alcohol with any medication, or when taking several drugs at the same time. Be sure to inform your doctor of any medication—prescription or nonprescription—you have been taking. Your pharmacist should also keep a record of all your prescriptions and over-the-counter drugs. This listing, generally called a Patient Drug Profile, is used to review your record should problems arise. You may want to keep your own record and bring it to your pharmacist for review whenever a new medicine is added.

Usual Dose: The maximum and minimum amounts of a drug that are usually prescribed. However, you may be given different dosage instructions by your doctor. It is important to check with your doctor if you are confused about how often to take a pill, and when, or if you have been given a dosage different from that indicated in this book. You should not change the prescribed dosage of any drug you are taking without first talking to your doctor.

Overdosage: The symptoms of a drug overdose and the immediate steps you should take if overdose occurs are detailed whenever there is a danger of an overdose reaction.

Certain drugs such as narcotic pain relievers (i.e., Percodan and Percocet) may cause you to become dependent or addicted to them. These pill profiles include additional sections on *Dependence and Addiction, Withdrawal Symptoms,* and *Withdrawal Treatment.*

If you read something in *The Pill Book of Arthritis* that does not coincide with your doctor's instructions, call your doctor. He may have had special reasons for prescribing different medications, or different dosages from those referred to here.

Any drug can have serious side effects if used improperly or abused. We advise you to learn all you can about the drugs you're taking—the benefits and dangers alike.

I
Arthritis in the 1980s

1.

WHAT IS ARTHRITIS?

Arthritis is a potentially serious illness. But in most cases, it doesn't have to limit your lifestyle. Of the 35 million people who require treatment for arthritic conditions, the great majority live comfortably—and actively—thanks to a growing understanding of the different diseases that collectively we call arthritis, and to increasingly sophisticated and effective treatment through the use of drugs, physiotherapy, and other means.

What does it mean when your doctor diagnoses arthritis? Technically, *arthron* means "joint" and *itis* signifies "inflammation." So, simply put, arthritis means that one or more of your joints is inflamed. But *arthritis,* as used by your doctor, is an umbrella term that covers over 100 separate and distinct diseases that involve factors from heredity and hormones to infection and injury. Some are not true joint inflammations, some occur in combination with other diseases, and almost all are perplexing, painful, and variable in their damage.

In order to understand the basic nature of some of the diseases that come under the "arthritis" umbrella, we can break them down into four major categories:

1. *Wear-and-tear arthritis.* (Most frequent) The deterioration of one or more parts of the joint is inevitable over time. When cartilage breaks down, for example, bones rubbing against each other can cause arthritic pain. Injuries, whether large and traumatic or small and recurring, will often hasten the onset of the destruction of a joint. As an accompaniment, the bones around the joint will grow thicker and become stiff. Wear-and-tear types of arthritis, such as osteoarthritis, can also involve inflammation.

2. *Inflammatory arthritis.* (Approximately one out of six arthritis sufferers) Inflammation is a natural process that occurs when body tissue is injured. Blood, and also special cells called inflammatory cells, rush to the injury site to fight, block, or destroy the effect of an irritant on body tissue. In the process, the congestion of blood and inflammatory cells in the affected area causes symptoms of redness, heat, swelling, pain, and immobilization of the area when nerve endings are compressed. All this is necessary and helpful in normal situations. But when inflammation becomes chronic, or occurs even when there is no obvious irritant, the process itself becomes harmful to the body. In these cases, such as that of rheumatoid arthritis, the natural healing process has "turned against" the body and is working to destroy it.

When this happens, the resulting arthritis is said to be caused by a defect in the body's immune system. For reasons that are unknown at present, the immune system begins to "fight" normal body tissue, causing inflammation, damage, and eventually destruction of the tissue.

3. *Arthritis caused by defects in body chemistry.* (Quite rare) Though these types of arthritis also involve inflammation, the cause is known, as in gout, for example. This type of arthritis will usually involve only one or two joints.

4. *Other types of arthritis.* (Approximately one out of five arthritis sufferers) Some types of arthritis are caused by or triggered by bacterial infection, such as staph arthritis or Reiter's syndrome. Less-common forms of arthritis have symptomatic inflammation as their common denominator.

Having one form of arthritis neither exempts you from having another type of arthritis nor points to the likelihood that you will. The only safe prediction is that you'll eventually develop some osteoarthritis.

Where Arthritis Begins

Arthritis is a disease of the joints. The joint, as a whole, is the area where two bones meet, usually to form a movable attachment, allowing the bending of knees and fingers, or walking and running. Every joint is an efficiently engineered piece of body machinery that consists of various parts, each with its own function. Arthritis causes pain by damaging or causing the disintegration of at least one of these parts:

• *Cartilage* prevents the two bone ends from rubbing against each other. Each bone end is coated with this tough, gristly material.

• The *synovial membrane* surrounds the joint and dispenses lubrication to ease bending and turning.

• The *joint capsule* surrounds the synovial

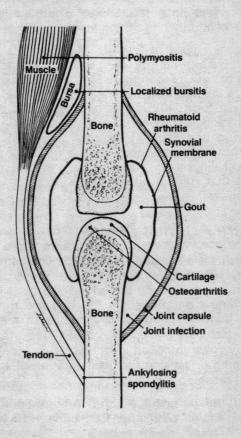

Sites of Arthritic Diseases

membrane and connects the two bones so that the joint remains stable.

• *Muscles,* which are usually found above or below a joint, turn into *tendons* where they attach to the bone.

• In some body parts, *bursae,* little sacs containing lubricating fluid, lie between the muscles and tendons in order to ease the movement of body tissues across each other. It is worth mentioning here that although the inflammation of the bursas may contribute to swelling around the joints in a disease such as rheumatoid arthritis, bursitis alone is fairly common and will most often subside without treatment. It is rarely necessary to resort to either cortisone treatment or surgery.

Although arthritis is primarily a disease of the joints, some forms of it are associated with inflammation of other body parts. These "associates" of arthritis can involve inflammation of the eyes, the skin, and even internal organs. Since these occur in conjunction with the arthritic process, they are considered symptoms of arthritis.

First Steps

What good will it do you to know these things? Plenty. As an arthritis patient, one of the first things you must know is how important it is for you to cultivate a good understanding of and good attitude about your arthritis. The medical world now agrees that a healthy, positive outlook has a positive impact on the success of your treatment. So, the more you know about your arthritis, the more in control you will feel, and the more able you will be to work with your doctor to beat your arthritis.

There is another important reason to educate

yourself on the subject: You, as an arthritis patient, have options. There are various forms of treatment. Some may be suitable for you; others may not be.

Read the following facts before you shrug and say, "It's only arthritis."

- *Arthritis is the nation's* number-one *crippling disease*
- *One-third of our nation—50 million people—have some form of arthritis*
- *7.5 million people are now disabled due to arthritis*
- *600,000 fall victim to arthritis each year— from infants to the elderly*
- *250,000 under age 16 are affected by juvenile rheumatoid arthritis*
- *15 million workdays are lost each year to arthritis*
- *$13 billion annually is spent for arthritis medical costs*
- *$5 billion each year goes for "quack" cures*

Source: Arthritis Foundation

Often it takes time and some amount of experimentation to arrive at the optimum treatment in your individual case. Though most doctors will be careful to let you know all possible drug side effects to watch for, and to warn you about levels of toxicity and the like, it's not enough to have only the memory of your doctor's explanation during your visit, and here's why: Anxiety runs high during a doctor's appointment—it's difficult to retain everything that is said and to retain it correctly. Chances are your doctor doesn't have the time to explain matters as fully as you would like. You may not understand what is being said, especially if you are unfamiliar with medical terms. Or you may hesitate to ask "dumb" questions.

In order to become a responsible patient, knowledgeable about helping yourself, you must know your disease and the treatments you will be taking for it.

2.

ARTHRITIS: MYTH AND REALITY

Arthritis has been with us since the very beginning. Neanderthal man had it; ancient Roman literature is full of references to gout and its sufferers; it has been said that Mary, Queen of Scots, had trouble climbing to her imprisonment in the Tower of London because of it. More recently, Katharine Hepburn, Sandy Koufax, and Gerald and Betty Ford are a few well-known personalities who have had various forms of this disease. How has arthritis been treated through the ages? "Cures" for arthritis, both ancient and modern, have been known to rival its symptoms. Take for example an ancient arthritis "cure" that required boiling wolves in oil and soaking in the broth! More-recent treatments have included sitting in uranium mines or taking snake venom or cocaine. And along with the myth that arthritis can be "cured" came many other myths that have erroneously become folk "wisdom." Here are some of the myths—and realities— about arthritis.

MYTH #1: Arthritis is a disease of old age.
REALITY: Arthritis can strike at *any* age, including infancy.

MYTH #2: There is nothing that can be done about arthritis.
REALITY: There are many things that can be done. Medication, if taken as directed, not only can affect the symptoms but can retard the progress of some forms of the disease. In some cases, physical therapy is extremely important and effective. Depending on your specific type of arthritis, a number of treatments and aids will help you overcome the disease.

MYTH #3: Having arthritis means drastic changes in the way you live.
REALITY: Dancers have it and still dance, athletes have it and still play—any number of people have it and continue to do things in their lives that are important to them. There are ways to "get around," "outsmart," or "live with" your arthritis that do not mean taking to your bed and waiting for "the end."

MYTH #4: Arthritis is a slow, progressive disease.
REALITY: Since arthritis is so many different diseases, it stands to reason that there are almost as many courses the disease can take. Depending on your heredity, your health, your attitude, and the type of arthritis you have, it may begin slowly, rapidly, or erratically; it may charge ahead, poke along, or come and go. Arthritis has been called a "disease of remission": you can't be sure when it will disappear completely or come back for a visit or to stay.

MYTH #5: Arthritis is not a serious disease.
REALITY: Because so many of us have a "touch of arthritis," it is not taken as seriously as it should be. Again, it is not one disease, but many different diseases, some of which can be *very* serious if left untreated.

MYTH #6: Diet is important in treating arthritis.
REALITY: Diet is an important factor in all our lives, but it is *not* more important for those who suffer from arthritis. Thus far, no link between diet and arthritis has been established in any form of arthritis with the exception of gout, and even that is treated more effectively with a specific drug— colchicine—than through dietary means.

MYTH #7: Aspirin is the only treatment, so save the doctor bills and treat yourself.
REALITY: Taking aspirin for arthritis is very different from taking two aspirin tablets every once in a while to ease minor pain. To be effective against inflammation, aspirin must be taken in high dosages, which may result in side effects. It is very important to be under a doctor's care. For those patients who cannot tolerate aspirin, there are many other drug possibilities. Therefore, it is both necessary and wise to work closely with your doctor to establish the best possible treatment regimen for your individual needs.

MYTH #8: There are alternative cures for arthritis— with proven results—that the medical world is either unaware of or refuses to recognize.
REALITY: No matter how much we'd like to think that quick and easy cures for arthritis exist and can be found, the truth is that most alternative treatment programs—those not under your doctor's

supervision—have no supportable basis in fact. The most popular of these alternative treatments are found in the box on page 21. But as a general guideline, here are three treatment categories to keep in mind: (1) those that can harm you; (2) those that neither help nor harm; and (3) those with limited or experimental use.

The first of these categories consists of treatments for arthritis that are not only ineffectual but that may do you harm. Leifcort, for example, a drug combination made popular in the 1960s, contains a steroid and is condemned by the FDA as "an irrational mixture of potent ingredients." Leifcort is still sold underground in the United States. Among the side effects suffered by its users are softening of the bones, high blood pressure, and cataracts.

The second category consists of those treatments that neither help nor harm. Most alternative treatment methods fall into this category, that of the "quack" cure. Arthritis is particularly susceptible to quackery because it is largely a disease of remission: that is, it seems to come and go for no apparent reason. A patient who is introduced to a new treatment and simultaneously undergoes remission will not know it wasn't due to the new "miracle" cure. Unfortunately, many testimonial-type advertisements are based on just such coincidences. If a medication has not been tested with consistent results by a number of reputable organizations over a long period of time, *there is no proof* that it is effective—and it probably is not. A well-informed patient with a questioning attitude will be able to spot the frauds, eliminate costly mistakes, and curb false hopes. Read medical journals, not tabloid papers, for factual information.

RATING ALTERNATIVE TREATMENTS

Here are some alternative arthritis treatments and how we rate them on our scale of helpfulness.

Potentially harmful

> *Bee stings*
> *Cocaine*
> *Flu shots*
> *Homeopathic medicine (i.e., arsenic, poison ivy)*
> *Leifcort, Rheumatril*
> *Mexican clinics*

Neither harmful nor helpful

> *Copper bracelets*
> *Climate*
> *Diet supplements (i.e., cod-liver oil, alfalfa)*
> *Mussel extract*
> *Pritikin Diet*
> *Vitamin, mineral supplements*

Of limited experimental use

> *Acupuncture*
> *Acupressure*
> *Biofeedback*
> *Cold and/or heat treatments*
> *Liniments, ointments, body rubs*
> *X-rays*

Although no immediate harm will come to you if you take noneffective cures like cod-liver oil or a climate change, such treatments can keep you going around in circles long enough to prevent your getting proper medical attention before your condition worsens or permanent damage occurs. This is probably the most harmful effect of "quack" cures. The time you waste could be spent refining the steps in a legitimate program designed to help you manage your disease. If you feel you must experiment in these areas, do so *in addition to* your regular treatment—and with the knowledge of your doctor.

Not *all* alternative methods are quackery. Some may even be cautiously approved by segments of the medical profession. This third category includes treatments with limited use, or ones that are still experimental. Biofeedback and acupuncture are two examples of treatment methods that may offer ways of controlling pain and discomfort. It is possible that such methods may be introduced as supplements to drug and other approved medical treatments.

Most doctors are well aware of the various treatments for arthritis, whether traditional or alternative. Specialists in particular keep up on the latest "popular" cures. Ask your doctor for information before you believe someone who may be trying to sell you a fake bill of goods.

3.

TYPES OF ARTHRITIS AND THEIR TREATMENT

Arthritis is a disease that takes many forms. It is essential for you to understand *which kind* of arthritis you have in order to treat it properly and live with it successfully.

Arthritic diseases in order of frequency:

Osteoarthritis

Rheumatoid arthritis

Ankylosing spondylitis

Systemic lupus erythematosus

Gout

Arthritis due to infection

Scleroderma

Rheumatoid Arthritis (RA)

This is the most common crippling form of arthritis. The cause of this disease is unknown, but the disease itself seems to be the source of the inflammation. It usually affects those in the 30–50-year-old age group. Women get it eight times more often than men. There is some evidence that there is a genetic predisposition to RA. Rheumatoid arthritis typically affects symmetrical joints: that is, if you have it in your left knee, you will probably have it in your right knee; if it's in your left hand, it will be in your right. There is no other disease in which body tissues suffer such prolonged and sustained inflammation.

The disease can take one of three courses: it can last a few months and leave no visible damage (monocyclic); it can come and go with periods of illness separated by periods of remission, usually without leaving permanent damage (polycyclic); or it can last for many years or even for life and can lead to serious impairment if not treated properly and early (chronic). Within any of these three courses of the disease, there may also be phases that range from acute, when the disease and discomfort are at their height, to remission, when the disease and subsequent pain and discomfort seem to disappear.

Symptoms

RA is characterized by joint pain and stiffness that are usually their worst in the mornings or after a period of inactivity. Inflammation is the hallmark of rheumatoid arthritis, with redness, swelling, and heat in the affected area or areas, often knuckles and toes first. If it starts in the fingers, the middle joints will usually be affected. RA affects the whole body, so the victim feels weak, listless, fatigued, loses appetite and weight, and may run a mild fever. RA may involve major body organs such as the eyes, heart, lungs, and muscles. Deformities may result as the joint becomes distorted from the swelling and destruction of the cartilage and loosening of the ligaments. Once the natural balance of the working parts is lost, the joint will lose function and muscles will weaken. Most common are deformities of the hands, feet, wrists, elbows, shoulders, and knees. It may eventually result in total disability. RA begins abruptly in about one out of ten cases.

Treatment

Drug treatment has been moderately successful in dealing with RA. Drugs may take anywhere from hours to months to take effect. The following are standard steps in the treatment of rheumatoid arthritis.

Aspirin

Aspirin is the treatment of choice of most doctors because it is both effective and relatively safe. It will reduce both pain and inflammation if taken in the right amounts. It is most frequently prescribed in large doses taken regularly for an indefinite period. Since large doses of aspirin may cause side effects, the patient must remain under close medical supervision. Some doctors have found acetaminophen (e.g., Tylenol) to be an anti-inflammatory agent (in large doses) as well as a painkiller.

But, if it can be tolerated, aspirin is probably the safest, least expensive, and most effective medication. The addition of antacids to some aspirin may be effective in aiding aspirin tolerance. For more information, see pp. 79, 92.

If aspirin cannot be tolerated, doesn't work, or for some other reason is not appropriate treatment, the next step is usually:

Nonsteroidal Anti-Inflammatory Drugs (NSAIDs)

Diflunisal (Dolobid); fenoprofen calcium (Nalfon); ibuprofen (Motrin); indomethacin (Indocin); meclofenamate sodium (Meclomen); mefenamic acid (Ponstel); naproxen (Naprosyn); oxyphenbutazone (Oxalid); phenylbutazone (Butazolidin); piroxicam (Feldene); sulindac (Clinoril); tolmetin sodium (Tolectin).

Like aspirin therapy, the treatment of RA with NSAIDs does nothing to suppress the fundamental disease process, but is what is called a "symptomatic therapy." NSAIDs are commonly prescribed for patients who cannot tolerate aspirin and are frequently found to be as effective, with less potential for harming the stomach lining and upper intestinal tract. They do have an advantage over aspirin in that fewer pills, over longer intervals of time, need to be taken. There are so many of these drugs on the market that it is impossible to call one distinctly more effective than another. It is very much an individual choice to be made between you and your doctor, depending on your reaction to each specific drug. *Because you build tolerance, many of these drugs lose their effectiveness with prolonged use, in which case others may then be substituted.* The NSAIDs profiled here are probably the ones most often prescribed, although new compounds are coming on the market regularly—so check with your doctor for the latest information on NSAIDs. For more information, see p. 81.

In the event that your arthritis does not respond satisfactorily to any of these, the next step would be:

Antimalarial Drugs

Although this family of drugs was developed for and is still used in the treatment of malaria, for unknown reasons they are effective in the reduction of inflammation in RA. These drugs accumulate slowly in the body and are slow to be eliminated, so their effects are long-lasting. Hydroxychloroquine (Plaquenil) is currently the most popular drug of the antimalarial class, since it is believed to cause fewer eye problems than other similar drugs. Your eyes should still be checked every six months, however. For more information, see pp. 87, 130.

Gold

Injected salts of gold are still considered the basic treatment of choice for the suppression of the fundamental disease process of RA. Approximately 70 percent of all patients receiving gold salts will experience benefits from the injections, which are given first at weekly intervals and later every two, three or even four weeks for an indefinite period. Unfortunately, 25–50 percent of patients will experience side effects—which is the main drawback to their use. For further details, see pp. 84, 122, 124.

Oral gold (under the generic name auranofin) is not on the market at the writing of this book. It is expected in a short time to supplant injected gold as the doctor's initial treatment of choice, since it appears to cause fewer side effects. For more information, see p. 85.

Penicillamine
(Cuprimine, Depen Titratabs)

Penicillamine has no relation to penicillin. Although this drug, taken by mouth, has been found to be as effective as injected gold in producing remission of RA, the number and severity of the side effects have made many doctors use this treatment with extreme caution. For those patients who have not responded to gold treatment or who cannot tolerate the side effects associated with gold, penicillamine has been used successfully in the treatment of severe RA. For more information, see pp. 86, 163.

Corticosteroids
(Cortisone, Prednisone, etc.)

These are the most potent of the anti-inflammatory drugs and produce dramatic improvement in the majority of RA patients. Their use in the treatment of this disease, or any other, is highly controversial, due to potentially serious side effects that can be expected with long-term use. Corticosteroid drugs can be given orally or by injection, or an injection of ACTH (a secretion of the anterior pituitary gland) can be given to stimulate the body's own production of adrenal cortical steroid hormone. *It is widely agreed that long-term oral treatment should be approached with great caution.*

Steroid joint injections should probably not exceed three or four shots per year in any joint.

Corticosteroids are available in both oral and injectable forms. Like the nonsteroidals, corticosteroids do not influence the course of the disease. For more information, see p. 82.

Immunosuppressives

In the continuing attempt to find a way to stop the body from destroying itself when the immune system has gone out of control, the role of immunosuppression is being explored. Only in the most extreme cases, and with the utmost caution, should this class of drugs be administered. For more information, see p. 86.

The immunosuppressive currently approved by the FDA for rheumatoid arthritis is azathioprine (Imuran). It is safer, though less effective, than cyclophosphamide (brand name Cytoxan—currently used experimentally for RA). Azathioprine has been approved for use in severe rheumatoid arthritis that is unresponsive to other conventional therapies. It is useful for those who cannot tolerate gold or penicillamine. It may alleviate the need for corticosteroids. For more information, see p. 96.

Physical Therapy

Physical therapy plays a major role in the treatment of the rheumatoid-arthritis patient. When applied during the acute phases of the disease, physical therapy is directed toward the soothing of inflammation by heat, rest, and gentle massage. During less-active periods it can retard the development of deformities and help restore function. Physical therapy, however, is most effective when drug therapy has been successful in suppressing the basic disease process. Physical therapy must be ordered by your doctor and carried out under medical supervision with regular follow-up.

Splinting

Splinting is the immobilization of a joint so that it can rest and heal. Particularly painful joints are sometimes helped by this enforced rest, but they should not remain immobile for too long. A splint may be worn only at night, for example. Even when a joint is splinted, it can be moved gently so that it doesn't become completely stiff. Splinting is frequently used to attempt to slow the development of certain hand deformities. The splint keeps the fingers in a normal position, but only when in place.

Orthopedic Surgery

Increasingly sophisticated orthopedic procedures have resulted in a great deal of relief of pain and significant improvement in joint function for patients with severe RA. Results are best when drug therapy has suppressed the basic disease process. Total joint replacement is probably the most successful procedure under these conditions, since there are no remnants of diseased tissue left. Hips and knees are by far the best candidates. Operations on the wrist, hand, and elbow areas have been less successful. Cosmetic results are sometimes more gratifying than functional ones in these areas. For advice on living with your arthritis and a look at future treatment possibilities, see chapters 4 and 6.

<u>*Prognosis*</u>

One in six patients with RA develops some crippling and deformity. RA can last anywhere from several months to many years. It can be one of the more depressing forms of arthritis, but it is also a type in which at least temporary remission is possible.

Juvenile Rheumatoid Arthritis (JRA)

Although arthritis in children is referred to as juvenile rheumatoid arthritis, there are actually a number of different forms, most of which differ from the adult form of RA. Most children afflicted with this disease have a good chance of complete recovery. Monoarticular, pauciarticular, or oligoarticular arthritis affect one or only a few joints. One of the forms of JRA is sometimes called Still's disease. This form of the disease is systemic, usually with little arthritic involvement. Polyarticular juvenile arthritis involves many joints and is more like true rheumatoid arthritis. Acute rheumatic fever usually follows strep throat and is actually an allergic reaction against the strep bacteria; it is not one of the specific forms of JRA.

Monoarticular juvenile arthritis affects the knee most frequently, but may affect other large joints that become swollen and sore. Eye problems may also occur.

Still's disease is characterized by very high fever, fatigue, muscle aches, and skin rash. The liver, speen, and lymph nodes may swell. An attack may last for days or weeks, then disappear. The disease can recur frequently or after an interval of years. The arthritis associated with Still's disease is usually mild to moderate, but may be severe.

Polyarticular juvenile arthritis usually affects children approaching adolescence. Many joints may become inflamed, as with RA. As with RA also, symmetrical joints are affected, usually wrists, knuckles, or knees.

Acute rheumatic fever which, again, is not a specific form of JRA but may include arthritis as a symptom, and may also include a heart murmur, fever, and skin rash. Different joints may be affected over the course of this disease, which is now rare. The arthritis that develops usually disappears in a few weeks.

Treatment

The approach to treatment of a JRA patient must be even more cautious than the normally conservative treatment procedure for adults with this disease. In many instances, not enough is known about what effect a course of treatment will have on young and growing bodies; in other instances, almost too much is known about the destruction and disability a course of treatment may provoke. Treatment of patients with JRA is defined more by what is not indicated than by what is.

Aspirin

Aspirin continues to be the favored treatment for JRA. Taken in anti-inflammatory doses, it has proven to be an effective treatment in most cases, and one whose side effects not only are tolerable but are not harmful to growth and development.

Nonsteroidal
Anti-Inflammatory Drugs (NSAIDs)

Diflunisal (Dolobid); fenoprofen calcium (Nalfon); ibuprofen (Motrin); indomethacin (Indocin); meclofenamate sodium (Meclomen); mefenamic acid (Ponstel); naproxen (Naprosyn); oxyphenbutazone (Oxalid); phenylbutazone (Butazolidin); piroxicam (Feldene); sulindac (Clinoril); tolmetin sodium (Tolectin).

NSAIDs, often used in the treatment of adults, are used more cautiously with children. Research into their potentially harmful effects on growth is still being conducted.

Corticosteroids
(Cortisone, Prednisone, etc.)

These are known to stop bone growth and to prevent children from reaching their normal adult height. For this reason, as well as the other dangerous aspects of corticosteroid use, extreme caution must be employed in using this treatment form. A short course of corticosteroids might be indicated only for a disease with acute symptoms, such as Still's disease, for example, or for severe eye problems. If corticosteriods are given every other day, their effect on retardation of growth is significantly lessened.

Antimalarial compounds, gold salts, and penicilla- mine are sometimes employed, but only with caution.

Physical therapy, swimming in particular, is often helpful. However, during disease activity, contact sports, like football, should be avoided.

Surgery is not often required in JRA, but an operation called capsulectomy, which releases soft tissue to increase motion, is sometimes performed.

Removal of joint fluid through a needle is rarely performed, as is **joint injection of corticosteroids,** which may speed up bone destruction.

Relief of stress may be another positive approach to the treatment of JRA that has, so far, gone untested. A study at the University of Rochester that explored the possibility of a link between JRA and emotional stress found that divorce, separation, the death of a parent, or other emotional traumas were part of the backgrounds of a significant number of JRA patients. Whether or not stress can be labeled a triggering factor is open to question. Stress reduction for children suffering from JRA, however, is an area of possible exploration.

Prognosis

The outlook for most of the forms of arthritis occurring in children is good to excellent. Two-thirds of children affected with JRA forms other than polyarticular juvenile arthritis recover completely and do not have arthritic problems as adults. Polyarticular-arthritis sufferers, however, have a less positive outlook. About one-half of children with this type of arthritis will continue to need treatment as adults.

Osteoarthritis (OA)

This is the type of "wear and tear" arthritis that almost everyone will eventually get. Because it is so common, particularly in those over age 50, many myths concerning arthritis are mistakenly based on osteoarthritis, also called "degenerative joint disease." More than one-half of those over 30 will have some symptoms of osteoarthritis. It is usually mild in nature, with little, if any, inflammation and no involvement of the immune system. It is associated with aging or an aftermath to injury such as dislocation or fracture. Osteoarthritis of the hands, hips, knees, neck, spine, and toes is especially common. In this disease, cartilage—the gristly material on the ends of bones—loses elasticity and deteriorates with age. Pain results when the two bone ends rub as the joint moves. In addition, the bones themselves may begin to change, growing thicker and developing bony lumps, which causes the area to become stiff and painful to move.

Symptoms

Osteoarthritis sufferers, in contrast to rheumatoid-arthritis sufferers, feel their worst at the end of the day, rather than in the morning. They may also feel worse after exercising. The disease is experienced as a dull ache or burning in the joints. The joints gradually stiffen. Most commonly affected are the base of the neck, the lower spine, the big toes, the knees and the hips. Joint pain and loss of function, especially in weight-bearing joints, is common. As the body attempts to repair itself in reaction to the wearing away of "old" cartilage and bone, new bone growths, called Heberden's nodes, often appear on the ends of joints of fingers. Initially this may cause prickling, redness, and tenderness, but these symptoms usually subside, leaving bony protrusions but no pain. Osteoarthritis of the spine can be totally incapacitating if the bony protrusions, called spurs, press against spinal nerves. In the legs, bony-growth pressure on the nerve root can cause pain down the back of the thigh and calf. Over a period of time this can lead to muscle weakness and loss of reflexes. This is one form of what is commonly known as sciatica.

In contrast to the symmetrical nature of rheumatoid arthritis, if osteoarthritis is found on one side of the body, it will not necessarily appear on the other. For example, if one hip is affected, the other may not be affected.

Osteoarthritis appears to be the result of combined genetic and hormonal influences, beginning frequently as female hormones decrease.

Treatment

Though the basic disease process of osteoarthritis is not particularly receptive to drug treatment, significant reduction of pain and inflammation can usually be accomplished with one of the following drugs.

Aspirin and Acetaminophen
(Datril, Tylenol, etc.)

In the treatment of osteoarthritis, these drugs function as analgesics, or pain relievers. The usual dosage is 2 regular-strength tablets every 4 hours as needed. Since there is little or no inflammation associated with this type of arthritis, it is unnecessary and ineffectual to take aspirin or acetaminophen in larger doses. For more information, see p. 79.

Nonsteroidal
Anti-Inflammatory Drugs (NSAIDs)

Diflunisal (Dolobid); fenoprofen calcium (Nalfon); ibuprofen (Motrin); indomethacin (Indocin); meclofenamate sodium (Meclomen); mefenamic acid (Ponstel); naproxen (Naprosyn); oxyphenbutazone (Oxalid); phenylbutazone (Butazolidin); piroxicam (Feldene); sulindac (Clinoril); tolmetin sodium (Tolectin).

These drugs are used most often in the treatment of osteoarthritis, particularly if aspirin cannot be tolerated or has not been effective. For more information, see p. 81.

Narcotic Pain Relievers

(Codeine with acetaminophen, codeine with aspirin, etc.)

These drugs are sometimes used for short-term relief of moderate to severe pain. It is important that you follow your doctor's orders carefully when taking these drugs. For more information, see p. 85.

Corticosteroids
(Cortisone, Prednisone, etc.)

On occasion, injections are given to patients with osteoarthritis with good effect, but usually the treatment is effective only when inflammation is present. Oral dosages of corticosteroids are not given for osteoarthritis.

Other Treatments

For osteoarthritis, physical measures are more important than drug treatment. A physiotherapy program including range-of-motion activities, such as swimming and walking and any other exercises that are smooth and gradual, has been found to be of most help. Regularity of exercise is important in strengthening the affected areas and maintaining mobility. In addition, bed rest, heat, and traction (for the spine) are important in making joints functional again. Once that is accomplished, regular exercise, proper body weight, and good health habits are essential.

In many cases, orthopedic surgery (especially of the hip) can produce excellent results. Devices and home aids such as canes or special can openers can also be extremely helpful.

Prognosis

The outlook for patients with osteoarthritis is relatively good. Crippling is a rarity; in fact, most osteoarthritis victims suffer few symptoms. Frequently the disease goes into remission for long periods or, at its worst, is slow to progress.

Gouty Arthritis

Called the "disease of kings," gout is the most painful form of arthritis and, some would argue, the most painful condition in all of medicine. Only a present-day gout sufferer can fully appreciate the torture that those afflicted with this disease went through in the past. Today, though there is still no cure for gout, there is a highly effective treatment that can control it. More than 1 million people in this country suffer from gout. They are almost exclusively men. The rare woman with gout is generally past menopause. Gout occurs when there is an excess of uric acid, a waste product, in the blood. Your uric acid level is influenced by heredity. Your body may actually overproduce uric acid (primary gout), or the kidneys may fail to eliminate uric acid from the bloodstream, frequently due to the use of diuretics (secondary gout). An excess of uric acid alone, however, does not cause a gout attack; only one person in ten with an elevated uric-acid level will develop it. In these persons, some unknown factor causes needlelike crystals of uric acid to form in the joint, leading to the irritation and inflammation of a gout attack.

Symptoms

Extraordinarily painful, this disease centers in the large joint of the big toe 75 percent of the time. However, it can occur in any joint, with the joint becoming hot, swollen, and excruciatingly tender. An advanced form, chronic tophaceous gout, is characterized by gritty deposits beneath the skin, usually near the joints, called tophi. If the condition is chronic, kidney stones—a form of gout— may develop.

Treatment

Thanks to medical science, the acute gout attack is a vanishing phenomenon. By lowering uric-acid levels in the blood, attacks can be prevented. Blocking of the inflammatory reaction can also be accomplished through drugs. The following drug treatments are most common for gout.

Colchicine

Apparently colchicine works by reducing the inflammatory response to gout crystals. Colchicine is not a pain reliever in the traditional sense, but it will relieve the pain of an acute gout attack if taken quickly at the recommended dose. It may also be taken to prevent gout attacks.

Nonsteroidal Anti-Inflammatory Drugs (NSAIDs)

Diflunisal (Dolobid); fenoprofen calcium (Nalfon); ibuprofen (Motrin); indomethacin (Indocin); meclofenamate sodium (Meclomen); mefenamic acid (Ponstel); naproxen (Naprosyn); oxyphenbutazone (Oxalid); phenylbutazone (Butazolidin); piroxicam (Feldene); sulindac (Clinoril); tolmetin sodium (Tolectin). For more information, see p. 81.

Uric-Acid-Lowering Drugs

Probenecid (Benemid), sulfinpyrazone (Anturane).

These drugs lower the uric-acid levels in the blood by promoting elimination of uric acid via the kidneys. Whether they are preferable to the following category of drugs described is a matter of controversy. For more information, see p. 83.

Drugs That Prevent Formation of Uric Acid

Allopurinol (Zyloprim, Lopurin).

Drugs in this category lower the amount of uric acid in the blood by preventing its formation, which eliminates kidney involvement.

Gout patients may be treated initially with colchicine after which they may be maintained indefinitely on uric-acid-lowering or formation-preventing drugs. If a patient shows a dramatic response to colchicine during the initial treatment, this is often called the Colchicine Therapeutic Test and confirms the doctor's diagnosis.

Diet and Gouty Arthritis

Though it is commonly believed that foods high in purine such as fatty meats and poultry, certain fish and shellfish and organ meats (kidneys, liver, and sweetbreads) can cause gout or that their elimination will cure it, no convincing evidence to support this belief has been found.

None of these foods is responsible for the disease, but all can worsen a condition, and should be eaten in moderation. In addition, drinking large amounts of water will aid in the elimination of the body's uric acid. Crash dieting may also bring on an attack since starvation causes a rise in uric acid. Gout cannot be treated through diet adjustment alone. Consult your doctor about combining diet with drug therapy for maximum results.

Alcohol, unlike the food categories mentioned, can have a definite and harmful effect on gout patients. Alcohol can bring on an attack and/or worsen a gout condition. Intake should be limited in consultation with your doctor.

Prognosis

Since the discovery of drugs that will control gout attacks, the outlook for victims of this disease is excellent. And, although dietary excess is *not* a major cause of gout, some foods may aggravate distress, alcohol in particular.

Pseudogout

A disease similar to gout, pseudogout occurs mostly in the later years of life. This form of arthritis differs from gout in two basic ways: First, the crystals in the joint space that cause irritation are not of uric acid but of somewhat less-painful calcium pyrophosphate. Second, treatment for pseudogout differs from treatment of true gout. In addition, pseudogout occurs most frequently in those over age 70 and affects women as often as it does men.

Symptoms

Intense pain and inflammation of one or more joints, usually the knee, often the wrists and ankles. Attacks may continue for long periods; sometimes the condition will appear to be chronic.

Treatment

Pseudogout does not respond to treatment as dramatically as does gout. The following drugs are the most effective in the majority of cases.

Corticosteroid Injections

Steroid injections directly into the joint may be effectively employed to ease pain in one area of the body for the short term. In fact, this is the treatment of choice. Since the duration of results varies with each patient, the advisability of continued treatment with steroid injections will be up to you and your doctor.

Nonsteroidal Anti-Inflammatory Drugs (NSAIDs)

Diflunisal (Dolobid); fenoprofen calcium (Nalfon); ibuprofen (Motrin); indomethacin (Indocin); meclofenamate sodium (Meclomen); mefenamic acid (Ponstel); naproxen (Naprosyn); oxyphenbutazone (Oxalid); phenylbutazone (Butazolidin); piroxicam (Feldene); tolmetin sodium (Tolectin).

These may have to be taken for prolonged periods. For more information, see p. 81.

Other Treatment

Physical therapy: It is best to have your physician or a physical therapist prescribe specific exercises for the affected joints.

Exercise: For the rest of your body, normal activities and exercises should be continued as regularly as possible. For more information, see p. 58.

Weight Control: This is especially important if weight-bearing joints are involved. See p. 58 for more detail.

Orthopedic Surgery: Knee or hip replacement rarely is needed, but can be performed when necessary. For more information, see p. 30.

Prognosis

Though sufferers of pseudogout may experience some degree of constant pain, the prognosis is generally good. Rarely does crippling result, and there is no serious threat to over-all health from the condition.

Ankylosing Spondylitis (AS)

Also called Marie-Strumpel disease, ankylosing spondylitis is a relatively rare disease that sometimes results in "poker spine," the complete inability to bend the spine. The name of this disease means literally "fused spine." It attacks men more often than women. It can occur at any age but tends most often to strike young adults. It is rare in blacks. AS usually affects the lower portion of the spine at the sacroiliac joint, where the spine joins the pelvic bone, but it can affect other joints of the spine. Hereditary predisposition is a major factor and can be traced to a genetic marker referred to as B-27. This disease destroys the joint or joints and gradually replaces them with connective tissue and then new bone, which is unbending and immovable.

Symptoms

Aching in one side of the buttocks, which soon moves to the other, and pain in the lower back, leg, or affected joint. Stiffness after immobility such as sleep or prolonged sitting. Swelling in knees or ankles. Low-grade fever, lassitude, and easy fatigue. Symptoms tend to come and go. Nighttime, when joints tend to stiffen, can be particularly painful. Some people have eventual loss of mobility of the spine and sometimes complete rigidity and curvature. Stooping posture may involve the neck as well as the back. Rib-to-spine fusion may also develop, resulting in breathing difficulty. Complications may include eye inflammation in 20–30 percent of victims.

Treatment

No drug will suppress or retard the development of deformities, but there are medications for relief of symptoms. Iritis (eye inflammation) usually responds to treatment. Physical therapy is the mainstay of treatment in this disease; a careful program should be worked out between you and your physical therapist. When properly carried out, physical therapy can prevent deformity and retard fusion, especially in the case of fusion of the ribs to the spine. Therapy treatment should be done two to three times per day for maximum benefit.

Anti-Inflammatory and Analgesic Drugs

These are given to relieve symptoms such as pain and immobility caused by swelling, so that the patient can carry out the physiotherapy program.

Prognosis

Ankylosing spondylitis most commonly occurs in very mild form with almost no physical consequences or disruption of life-style. Only one in one hundred patients develops serious deformity.

Reiter's Syndrome

Reiter's syndrome, like AS, usually affects young men. It is linked with AS because of the characteristics the two diseases have in common—the genetic marker B-27 and the population they strike most often. The inflammation of Reiter's syndrome involves both eye and urinary-tract as well as large-joint arthritis and Achilles-tendon inflammation. It may be associated with ulcerative colitis, regional enteritis, and psoriasis. Infection seems to be the cause of Reiter's syndrome, usually following either sexual exposure or severe cases of diarrhea.

Symptoms

Spinal pain and stiffness; heel pain; conjunctivitis or other eye inflammation; discharge from the urethra; skin rash on the palms of hands or soles of feet. Frequently involves only one side of the body. Usually comes in cycles; each may last several weeks to several months.

Treatment

This disease can be difficult to treat, and it may respond to anti-inflammatory agents differently at different times. The following are the most common drug treatments.

Nonsteroidal Anti-Inflammatory Drugs (NSAIDs)

Diflunisal (Dolobid); fenoprofen calicum (Nalfon); ibuprofen (Motrin); indomethacin (Indocin); melcofenamate sodium (Meclomen); mefenamic acid (Ponstel); naproxen (Naprosyn); oxyphenbutazone (Oxalid); phenylbutazone (Butazolidin); piroxicam (Feldene); tolmetin sodium (Tolectin).

These may have to be taken for prolonged periods. For more information see pg. 81.

Immunosuppressives

Azathioprine: This immunosuppressive is only rarely used for severe cases that have not responded to other treatment. Side effects include lowered resistance to infection and possible risk of cancer. Blood tests are required regularly. Never take this drug with allopurinol (Lopurin, Zyloprim), as the two drugs combined can be fatal. For more information, see pp. 86, 96.

Methotrexate: Again, this immunosuppressive is employed as treatment only in the most severe cases. Though effective, the side effects of liver damage, lowered resistance to infection, and possible cancer make it a highly undesirable choice. Blood tests are required regularly.

Other Treatment

Physical therapy: Range-of-motion exercises are most frequently recommended.

Rest: A combination of exercise and rest of the affected joints should be discussed with your doctor or physical therapist.

Prognosis

The disease is alternately active and inactive. It often does not result in crippling, but it may. Associated eye problems must be treated seriously to prevent loss of sight.

Systemic Lupus Erythematosus (SLE)

Lupus, as it is called, is not a true arthritis but is linked with arthritis about 50 percent of the time. Lupus, meaning "wolf," refers to the rash that commonly covers the victim's cheeks and nose. Lupus is one of the most serious of the arthritis-associated diseases. It can involve many vital internal organs, especially the kidneys. In rare instances it may be fatal. Like rheumatoid arthritis, it occurs primarily in women and young girls—five times more often than in men. It usually develops in young adulthood. Often, victims also have Raynaud's disease—the blanching or mottling of the hands and feet upon exposure to cold, which disappears after warming. Lupus occurs when antibodies created by the body attack other parts of the body. In effect, the body is fighting itself. In lupus-associated arthritis, the body uses its own defense system to attack the lining of the joints.

Symptoms

The joint symptoms of lupus are in many ways identical to RA. Lupus may be present for years before it is apparent. Other symptoms of lupus depend on the area or areas of the body under attack. Lupus may involve such vital organs as the kidneys, which may result in hypertension and generalized body swelling. Central nervous system disease results in psychosis, bizarre behaviour, or epileptic seizures. Heart involvement produces chest pain or irregular heartbeat. Other symptoms may include bleeding gums or excessive menstrual bleeding. The only specific known cause of flareups is exposure to sunlight. Suitable precautions and sun-screens should be used to screen ultraviolet light.

Treatment

The treatment of lupus relies largely on drugs that reduce inflammation or decrease the amount of abnormal antibodies produced, such as the following.

Corticosteroids
(Cortisone, Prednisone, etc.)

Although the use of corticosteroids in the treatment of most diseases associated with arthritis is not often recommended, the seriousness of some forms of SLE can be good reason to employ them. In some cases, high doses of these drugs have been found to arrest normally fatal lupus kidney disease and other life-threatening manifestations of lupus. With proper dosage and duration of treatment, inflammation and consequent damage to internal organs can be suppressed until the natural remission of the disease. Although the side effects are distressing and dangerous, the consequences of leaving this serious disease untreated are more so. For more information, see p. 82.

Immunosuppressives
(Azathioprine, Cytoxan, Chlorambucil)

These drugs are not officially indicated for the treatment of lupus. However, they are sometimes used in combination with steroids and are believed to lessen the need for steroids in some cases. Careful supervision is required, however, since these drugs have their own unique profile of side effects, the most dangerous of which is the lowering of the body's resistance to infection.

Rest

As with all tissue connective disease, rest can be an important part of the overall treatment of lupus. Flare-ups may be traced to stress caused by overwork, emotional pressures, and other environmental factors. Rest and relaxation can result in improved conditions.

<u>Prognosis</u>

Arthritis associated with lupus only rarely causes crippling, although it may remain active over a long period of time. Prognosis for patients with lupus depends on the type they have but can generally be said to be good, particularly with effective drug therapy.

Progressive Systemic Sclerosis (Scleroderma)

Scleroderma means literally "thickening of the skin." It is not a true arthritis but rather a disease that involves thickening of the body's connective tissue, with accompanying symptoms of arthritis. Scleroderma affects more women than men and usually occurs between the ages of 40 and 60. It was believed at first to affect only the skin, hence the name, but it was later found to affect vital internal organs as well. For unknown reasons, the body gives the "repair" signal when there is no significant inflammation. This repair mechanism goes out of control and continues to produce collagen at an accelerated rate, depositing increased amounts of connective tissue on the affected area or areas. This decreases the blood supply available to tissues, and they starve. Gradually, dense, fibrous tissue replaces normal elastic skin structures. When this growth is over vital organs, it can be life threatening. For example, kidney involvement can result in potentially dangerous high blood pressure or kidney failure. Often Raynaud's disease— the blanching or mottling of the hands and feet upon exposure to cold, which disappears when warm—accompanies scleroderma.

Symptoms

One or more of the following symptoms may be present. Thickening of the skin anywhere on the body—usually the fingers, forearms, face, and neck—characterizes this disease. There may be mild joint inflammation and loss of joint mobility (i.e., tightening of the skin over fingers, elbows, knees, etc.). Calcium deposits are sometimes found under the skin, along with red spots (called telangiectasia). Hair growth may stop, and there may be intense itching or ulceration of the skin over the fingertips and the joints, or loss of finger length. If there is thickening of the skin over the chest wall, breathing is imparied and there may be decreased oxygen in the blood, heart failure, and fluid accumulation in the legs. If the growth is in the esophagus, there may be difficulty in swallowing, pain under the breastbone, hyperacidity (heartburn), and esophagitis. Intestinal malabsorption can lead to semistarvation. Kidney involvement may be signaled by severe hypertension in addition to protein in the urine, seizures, decreased vision, and loss of kidney function.

Treatment

There is no cure for scleroderma. The drugs used in treatment can help only in coping with problems resulting from specific organ involvement.

Antihypertensive Drugs

Preliminary research has shown that in patients with PSS, prolonged reduction of high blood pressure and kidney involvement may produce an improvement in the sclerodermatous condition of the skin.

Corticosteroids
(Cortisone, Prednisone, etc.)

These should be used with caution and for the shortest time possible in the treatment of inflammation of muscles when complications in the disease occur.

Immunosuppressives
(Azathioprine, Chlorambucil)

These are an extremely potent—and, thus far, experimental—approach to the treatment of PSS. Recommended only in the most severe cases.

There are, of course, many other drugs used to treat specific manifestations of PSS. Here we deal only with the connective tissue involvement of the disease.

Other Treatment

Therapeutic exercise: Active exercise to stretch the skin, to make the most use of the joints, and to improve circulation should be repeated several times a day. Consult your doctor or physical therapist to help you devise a program suited to your needs.

Attitude: More than most diseases, PSS can be affected positively by a good mental outlook, which can serve to increase blood flow through narrowed vessels.

Biofeedback is another method that has been used to help overcome scleroderma through improving blood circulation.

<u>*Prognosis*</u>

The outlook for this disease, despite the extreme-sounding symptoms, is generally good. Scleroderma usually runs its course in two years or less, with improvement often occurring afterward. Less than 10 percent of scleroderma patients develop the most serious type of this disease, which involves kidney problems.

Other Forms of Arthritis

Arthritis Due to Infection

This is the only curable type of arthritis. There are a number of different bacterial infections that can affect a joint, including staphylococcus (the most serious), meningitis, gonorrhea, pyelonephritis (infection of the kidney), infections of the gallbladder and lungs, tuberculosis, and osteomyelitis. One type, the recently discovered Lyme arthritis (named for the Connecticut town where it was first diagnosed), is caused by the bacteria transported by a particular kind of tick.

Various kinds of bacteria may be passed from the bloodstream into the joint space, where they cause an acute reaction leading to the formation of pus and possible destruction of the joint.

Depending on the type of infection, time can be a pivotal factor. Joints can be destroyed in a matter of days, or the infection can lead to chronic degenerative arthritis if not treated in time. Damage to joints cannot be undone, and joints previously damaged by arthritis disease are particularly susceptible. In some cases, there can also be involvement of the brain, heart and other internal organs.

Symptoms

Each infection may present its own range of symptoms, including arthritis. Initially, arthritis may not be a major concern; in Lyme arthritis, for example, a rash around the tick bite is usually followed by flu-like symptoms, and arthritis develops only weeks later. However, any of these infections may result in serious damage and should not be ignored.

Treatment

Depending on the type of germ, there are various antibiotic drugs that will usually cure arthritis caused by a bacterial infection.

Prognosis

If medical help is sought promptly, most types of infectious arthritis can be cured. Without treatment, staphylococcal infection is fatal. Once treated, the arthritis caused by infection usually clears up, leaving no permanent damage.

Other less-common forms of arthritis are linked by symptomatic inflammation.

Psoriatic Arthritis

It is not widely known that this common skin condition is directly related to specific types of arthritis. See Reiter's disease and AS.

Dermatomyositis, Polymyositis

Not true arthritis, these are systemic diseases of the skin and muscles near joints, causing muscular weakness and destruction.

Vasculitis

Again, not a true arthritis, this disease involves inflammation of the blood vessels, the arteries, and the veins.

Polyarteritis

Literally "inflammation of many arteries," a form of vasculitis, this is the most serious type of blood-vessel inflammation.

4.

LIVING WELL WITH ARTHRITIS

There is every reason for the person with arthritis to lead an active, satisfying life. With your doctor's approval and guidance, your present activities need not change, but may need only modification once your individualized program of treatment is established. Remember, though, that whatever your treatment program is, it may take a number of months before results can be expected.

Work

An estimated 90 percent of people with arthritis are employable. Depending on the type of arthritis you have and the joints it affects, you may have to be selective about the work you do. If your arthritis involves the joints of your fingers, a typing job is not for you. But by using your common sense you will be able to remain useful, productive, and independent.

Exercise

Swimming is probably the best exercise for arthritis, preferably in a heated pool. Joints are kept flexible without undergoing undue stress. Isometric and range-of-motion exercises that put the joints of the body through their full range of movement are also favored by doctors, as long as such exercises do not increase pain. When you hit a trouble spot, stop, but keep going back until you are gradually able to increase your range of motion without pain. Your doctor may recommend either physical therapy or a consultation with a physical therapist to design an exercise program appropriate for you. In general, activities that do not cause aching, stiffness, or pain are recommended.

Diet and Weight Control

If you are overweight, a low-calorie diet is strongly recommended so that excess weight does not increase the strain on joints. This is particularly important if any weight-bearing joints are involved in your arthritis. If your weight is normal, a well-balanced diet is recommended, with vitamin supplements as needed. There is no proof that diet is related to any form of arthritis with the exception of gout, and even that disease is best treated with drug therapy. Eating sensibly will go further to help your condition than any "arthritis" diet that has no basis in fact.

Rest

An often ignored area of treatment, rest can be surprisingly effective in the treatment of various types of arthritis. Rest is required particularly when joint inflammation is active. During an acute phase of rheumatoid arthritis, for example, you might require complete bed rest, although you would still want to repeat simple movements several times a day to ward off stiffness. But rest should also be included in your daily routine. It can be every bit as healing as exercise, diet, and sometimes even medicine, and should be recognized and included in most treatment programs.

Sex

There are both physical and emotional elements involved in any discussion of sex. The physical problems experienced by arthritis sufferers are probably the most easily handled. It is true that, depending on the form of arthritis and the joints affected, discomfort or pain may be experienced during sexual intercourse. However, there are ways that discomfort can be minimized. Experiment with vaginal lubricants, warm baths, pillows under sensitive areas, and different positions. Ask your doctor for suggestions, too. This is an area of your life that may require some thoughtful change, but chances are you will be able to adapt.

The emotional aspects of the problem are harder to deal with since they involve not reality, but one's ego. Perhaps you don't feel as attractive as you used to or as confident. Again, these are topics to discuss with your doctor or perhaps a psychological consultant. Just as you would seek physical therapy, emotional therapy may be part of an overall treatment program to help you function at your best.

Another possibility is that the drug treatment you are undergoing may be responsible for a decrease in your sexual appetite, or that the side effects are disturbing enough to interfere. In either case, inform your doctor of your difficulty. Your doctor will probably consider adjusting the dosage or changing your medication entirely.

Fatigue associated with arthritis is often another cause for a decrease in sexual activity. This can sometimes be avoided if you are able to readjust your schedule so that lovemaking occurs at times when you are feeling your best.

In any event, this is a vital area of life, whatever your age or condition. As with other facets of your life with arthritis, confront the problem, then work out the best solution possible, with as much help as you can get.

Transfer Problems

If you find yourself having to "flop" into a chair in order to sit down, or to "rock" your body to stand up, you have a transfer problem. The "flop and rock" method is dangerous and could result in a very serious fall. A few simple modifications will lessen the chances of your falling.

• Raise chairs with cushions or wooden blocks.
• Attach a grab bar to the wall nearest the toilet, or to the toilet itself.
• If your knees are stiff or weak, raise your bed 2 to 4 inches.
• To improve your ability to get in and out of bed, use a firm mattress and headboard.
• Attach a sturdy cord or belt to the headboard or to other nearby secure fixtures, such as a radiator, to help you get in and out of bed.

Walking

Not everyone who has arthritis has difficulty getting around. However, if you find walking difficult, consider the following tips.

- If your legs are weak, or if you have a balance problem, a standard pickup walker may be useful.
- People with wrist, elbow, or hand problems may modify their walkers with platform attachments.
- Wheels, with autostops, may be attached to the walker if you have trouble lifting it.
- A cane is useful when one side of the body is afflicted.
- A cane should always be used on the side *opposite* the most painful or afflicted areas.
- In most cases, a properly adjusted walking aid results in the user's elbows being straight.
- Periodically check all bolts and rubber tips on walking aids.

Falls

Some arthritis sufferers are vulnerable to falls because their afflicted joints restrict their ability to step over objects. Following are some suggestions to help eliminate falling.

- Secure or remove scatter rugs.
- Place telephone cords and electrical wires behind heavy furniture or rugs.
- Improve lighting to make objects easier to spot.
- Tape edges of steps with reflective tape.

Bathing

If your arthritis prevents you from bathing, consider these tips.

- Install a railing alongside the bathtub.
- Install a shower seat.

• Use a spray hose with an extension to help reach all areas of your body.

• Place skid strips in the tub.

Home Aids

Many home aids can be used to make telephone dialing and kitchen work easier. The telephone company offers push-button phones with large, easy-to-read numbers. Or you may want a

---

ARTHRITIS DO's AND DON'T's

Do *maintain good posture, whether you are walking, standing, or sitting. Never slouch.*

Do *interrupt any sustained physical activity with a short rest period every ten to fifteen minutes.*

Do *make time for recommended exercises every day. Don't consider regular daily activities to be part of your exercise program.*

Do *push an object instead of pulling it. Use your leg muscles rather than straining your arms. Push with the palms of your hands instead of pushing with your fingers.*

Do *sit to work. Sitting reduces strain on your joints and saves energy. Work surfaces often can be adjusted to convenient heights.*

Do *avoid everyday actions that tend to promote discomfort. For example, a woman should use a purse that can be carried on the shoulder or arm rather than one that must be carried with the fingers.*

Do *dress appropriately for the weather. Although cold and damp have no direct bear-*

phone system that allows prerecorded numbers to be dialed with the push of one button.

If you have a hard time grabbing small objects, you can obtain devices made especially for people with arthritis. In fact, in one recent study, people with arthritis reported that these home aids were of greater benefit to them than anything else, including their medication. Please contact your local Arthritis Foundation for more information regarding home aids.

---

ing on your disease, they can make your aches and pains worse if you are not protected properly.

Don't *keep any joint in one position for too long. Don't sit for more than twenty minutes without moving.*

Don't *fall heavily into a chair. Lower yourself into the chair gently. And when you stand up, use the arms of the chair to help you rise slowly.*

Don't *put too much stress on vulnerable finger joints. Avoid opening jars with your hands. Use a jar opener.*

Don't *use tools with small grips. Use tools with large, wide handles.*

Don't *sleep with pillows under your knees or neck. The joints may stiffen in the bent position and be difficult to straighten in the morning.*

Don't *pull bed sheets or blankets tightly over your feet. This will interfere with circulation.*

Source: The Arthritis Foundation

If you're out to beat your arthritis and maintain a healthy, happy, active life, there are people, books, and organizations who want to help you. What you can do for yourself is be curious, stay informed, and maintain a positive outlook. The following are places to start your search for information and inspiration.

Dressing

If you have a hard time getting dressed, especially with your shoes, socks, or stockings, you may find long-handled shoe horns, elastic shoe laces, or velcro bindings helpful.

Chapters & Divisions of The Arthritis Foundation

ALABAMA
Alabama Chapter
13 Office Park Circle,
 Rm 14
Birmingham, AL 35223
Tel: (205) 870-4700

South Alabama Chapter
304 Little Flower Avenue
Mobile, AL 36606
Tel: (205) 471-1725

ARIZONA
Central Arizona Chapter
2102 W. Indian School
 Rd., Suite 9
Phoenix, AZ 85015
Tel: (602) 264-7679

Southern Arizona Chapter
4520 E. Grant Road
Tuscon, AZ 85712
Tel: (602) 326-2811

ARKANSAS
Arkansas Chapter
6213 Lee Avenue
Little Rock, AR 72205
Tel: (501) 664-7242

CALIFORNIA
Northeastern California
 Chapter
1722 "J" St., Suite 321
Sacramento, CA 95814
Tel: (916) 446-7246

Northern California
  Chapter
203 Willow St.
Suite 201
San Francisco, CA 94107
Tel: (415) 673-6882

San Diego Area Chapter
6154 Mission Gorge
  Rd., Suite 110
San Diego, CA 92120
Tel: (619) 280-0304

Southern California
  Chapter
4311 Wilshire Boulevard
Los Angeles, CA 90010
Tel: (213) 938-6111

COLORADO
Rocky Mountain Chapter
234 Columbine St.,
  Suite 210
P.O. Box 6919
Denver, CO 80206
Tel: (303) 399-5065

CONNECTICUT
Connecticut Chapter
370 Silas Deane Highway
Wethersfield, CT 06109
Tel: (203) 563-1177

DELAWARE
Delaware Chapter
234 Philadelphia Pike,
  Suite 1
Wilmington, DE 19809
Tel: (302) 764-8254

DISTRICT OF COLUMBIA
Metropolitan Washington
  Chapter
2424 Pennsylvania Ave.,
  N.W. Room #105
Washington, D.C. 20037
Tel: (202) 331-7395

FLORIDA
Florida Chapter
3205 Manatee Ave. West
Bradenton, FL 33505
Tel: (813) 748-1300

GEORGIA
Georgia Chapter
2799 Delk Road, S.E.
Marietta, GA 30067
Tel: (404) 952-4254
Toll Free: 1-800-282-7023

HAWAII
Hawaii Chapter
200 North Vineyard,
  Suite 505
Honolulu, HI 96817
Tel: (808) 523-7561

IDAHO
Idaho Chapter
700 Robbins Rd., Suite 1
Boise, ID 83702
Tel: (208) 344-7102

ILLINOIS
Central Illinois Chapter
Allied Agencies Center
320 East Armstrong Ave.,
  Rm 102
Peoria, IL 61603
Tel: (309) 672-6337

Illinois Chapter
79 W. Monroe,
   Suite 1120
Chicago, IL 60603
Tel: (312) 782-1367

INDIANA
Indiana Chapter
1010 East 86th Street
Indianapolis, IN 46240
Tel: (317) 844-3341

IOWA
Iowa Chapter
1501 Ingersoll Ave.,
   Suite 101
Des Moines, IA 50309
Tel: (515) 243-6259

KANSAS
Kansas Chapter
1602 East Waterman
Wichita, KS 67211
Tel: (316) 263-0116

KENTUCKY
Kentucky Chapter
1381 Bardstown Road
Louisville, KY 40204
Tel: (502) 459-6460

LOUISIANA
Louisiana Chapter
4700 Dryades
New Orleans, LA 70115
Tel: (504) 897-1338

MAINE
Maine Chapter
37 Mill Street
Brunswick, ME 04011
Tel: (207) 729-4453

MARYLAND
Maryland Chapter
12 West 25th Street
Baltimore, MD 21218
Tel: (301) 366-0923

MASSACHUSETTS
Massachusetts Chapter
59 Temple Place
Boston, MA 02111
Tel: (617) 542-6535

MICHIGAN
Michigan Chapter
23400 Michigan Ave.,
   Suite 605
Dearborn, MI 48124
Tel: (313) 561-9096

MINNESOTA
Minnesota Chapter
122 West Franklin,
   Suite 440
Minneapolis, MN 55404
Tel: (612) 874-1201

MISSISSIPPI
Mississippi Chapter
6055 Ridgewood Road
Jackson, MS 39211
Tel: (601) 956-3371

MISSOURI
Eastern Missouri Chapter
4144 Lindell Boulevard
St. Louis, MO 63108
Tel: (314) 533-1324

Western Missouri–
Greater Kansas City
   Chapter
8301 State Line,
   Suite 117
Kansas City, MO 64114
Tel: (816) 361-7002

MONTANA
Montana Chapter
100 West 24th Street
Billings, MT 59102
Tel: (406) 652-1538

NEBRASKA
Nebraska Chapter
120 North 69th Street,
   Rm 202
Omaha, NB 68132
Tel: (402) 558-2400

NEVADA
Nevada Division
2700 State Street, Suite
   14A
Las Vegas, NV 89109
Tel: (702) 369-8102

NEW HAMPSHIRE
New Hampshire Chapter
P.O. Box 369
35 Pleasant Street
Concord, NH 03301
Tel: (603) 224-9322

NEW JERSEY
New Jersey Chapter
15 Prospect Lane
Colonia, NJ 07067
Tel: (201) 388-0744

NEW MEXICO
New Mexico Chapter
5112 Grand Avenue,
   N.E.
Albuquerque, NM 87108
Tel: (505) 265-1545

NEW YORK
Central New York
   Chapter
505 E. Fayette Street,
   2nd Floor
Syracuse, NY 13202
Tel: (315) 422-8174

Genesee Valley Chapter
973 East Avenue
Rochester, NY 14607
Tel: (716) 271-3540

Long Island Division
501 Walt Whitman Road
Melville, NY 11747
Tel: (516) 427-8272

New York Chapter
115 East 18th Street
New York, NY 10003
Tel: (212) 477-8310

Northeastern New York
   Chapter
1237 Central Avenue
Albany, NY 12205
Tel: (518) 459-5082

Western New York Chapter
1370 Niagara Falls Blvd.
Tonawanda, NY 14150
Tel: (716) 837-8600

NORTH CAROLINA
North Carolina Chapter
P.O. Box 2505
3115 Guess Road
Durham, NC 27705
Tel: (919) 477-0286

NORTH DAKOTA
Dakota Chapter
1402 North 39th Street
Fargo, ND 58102
Tel: (701) 282-3653

OHIO
Central Ohio Chapter
2501 N. Star Road
Columbus, OH 43221
Tel: (614) 488-0777

Northeastern Ohio Chapter
11416 Bellflower Road
Cleveland, OH 44106
Tel: (216) 791-1310

Northwestern Ohio
   Chapter
4447 Talmadge Road
Toledo, OH 43623
Tel: (419) 473-3349

Southwestern Ohio
   Chapter
2400 Reading Road
Cincinnati, OH 45202
Tel: (513) 721-1027

OKLAHOMA
Eastern Oklahoma Chapter
2816 East 51st. Suite 120
Tulsa, OK 74105
Tel: (918) 743-4526

Oklahoma Chapter
3313 Classen Blvd.,
   Suite 101
Oklahoma City, OK 73118
Tel: (405) 521-0066

OREGON
Oregon Chapter
Barbur Blvd. Plaza
4445 S.W. Barbur Blvd.
Portland, OR 97201
Tel: (503) 222-7246

PENNSYLVANIA
Central Pennsylvania
   Chapter
P.O. Box 668
2019 Chestnut Street
Camp Hill, PA 17011
Tel: (717) 763-0900

Eastern Pennsylvania
   Chapter
311 So. Juniper St.,
   Suite 201
Philadelphia, PA 19107
Tel: (215) 735-5272

Western Pennsylvania
   Chapter
2201 Clark Building
Pittsburgh, PA 15222
Tél: (412) 566-1645

RHODE ISLAND
Rhode Island Chapter
850 Waterman Avenue
East Providence, RI 02914
Tel: (401) 434-5792

SOUTH CAROLINA
South Carolina Chapter
1802 Sumter St.
Columbia, SC 29201
Tel: (803) 254-6702

SOUTH DAKOTA
See North Dakota

TENNESSEE
Middle-East Tennessee
  Division
1719 West End Bldg.,
  Suite 619
Nashville, TN 37203
Tel: (615) 329-3431

West Tennessee Chapter
2600 Poplar Ave.,
  Suite 200
Memphis, TN 38112
Tel: (901) 452-4482

TEXAS
North Texas Chapter
5415 Maple Ave.,
  Suite 417
Dallas, TX 75235
Tel: (214) 638-7474

Northwest Texas Chapter
3145 McCart Avenue
Fort Worth, TX 76110
Tel: (817) 926-7733

South Central Texas
  Chapter
503 South Main Street
San Antonio, TX 78204
Tel: (512) 224-4857

Texas Gulf Coast Chapter
9099-A Katy Freeway
Houston, TX 77024
Tel: (713) 468-6572

West Texas Chapter
2317 34th St.
Lubbock, TX 79410
Tel: (806) 747-5125

UTAH
Utah Chapter
Graystone Plaza #15
1174 E. 2700 South
Salt Lake City, UT 84106
Tel: (801) 486-4993

VERMONT
Vermont Chapter
215 College Street
Burlington, VT 05401
Tel: (802) 864-4988

VIRGINIA
Virginia Chapter
1900 Byrd Ave., Suite 100
P.O. Box 6772
Richmond, VA 23230
Tel: (804) 282-5491

WASHINGTON
Western Washington
  Chapter
726 Broadway,
  Suite 103
Seattle, WA 98122
Tel: (206) 324-9940

WEST VIRGINIA
West Virginia Chapter
P.O. Box 8473
440 Fourth Avenue
South Charleston,
  WV 25303
Tel: (304) 744-3042

WISCONSIN
Wisconsin Chapter
1442 N. Farwell Ave.,
  Suite 508
Milwaukee, WI 53202
Tel: (414) 276-0490
Toll Free: 1-800-242-9945

WYOMING
See Colorado

5.

YOU AND YOUR DOCTOR

Nobody's perfect. Not you, not your doctor. But by keeping in mind these ten ways to become a successful patient, you'll help yourself get the best possible care for whatever type of arthritis you have.

1. **Admit to yourself that you have the disease.** Don't deny that there is something wrong with you if all the evidence points in the other direction. The first step in solving *any* problem is admitting it's there.

2. **Visit your doctor as instructed.** With many of the arthritic diseases, absence of pain does not necessarily mean that damage is not occurring in your body. Go to your doctor even if you are feeling better. Once you have placed yourself under a doctor's care, you have a responsibility as a patient to cooperate in your treatment.

3. **Take your medication as prescribed.** The best medicine in the world can't do any good if it isn't taken. And it can, in fact, do harm if it is not taken properly.

4. **Monitor your reaction to the medication prescribed.** Your doctor cannot know how you might react to certain medications unless he or she has your complete medical history, including drugs you have taken in the past and your reactions to them. Even so, it is wise for you to monitor your reactions to the medications prescribed by your doctor. Side effects can range from mild to severe, but each should be reported so that dosages can be adjusted, or so that you can be taken off any medication before a reaction becomes serious.

5. **Raise your consumer consciousness.** This book provides factual information about every approved drug for the treatment of arthritis. What it cannot do is prevent individuals or certain drug manufacturers from presenting you with misleading information. If you become aware of various techniques that are used to sell products from pills to "Magic Massage Mittens," you will be less likely to be a victim of the $1 billion per year arthritis-cure fraud. Don't be a sitting duck for a quack.

6. **Keep a record of medications you are taking or have taken in the past.** If you are seeing a new doctor, or change doctors in the future, this will save time and trouble and will help avoid mistakes. Include dosages and side effects you experienced as well as the reason why the medication was prescribed and how long you took it.

7. **When you visit a doctor for the first time, be prepared to give a complete family medical history.** Write down as much as you can in advance, including conditions and diseases you or your immediate family members (grandparents, parents, siblings) have or have had.

8. **Become an ally to your doctor.** Help assess your condition by being able to describe symp-

toms simply and concisely. Maintain a positive outlook—studies now prove that this actually helps in your treatment. Keep an open mind—don't decide what is wrong with you and then shop for a doctor who will agree.

9. **Flexible mind, flexible body.** Be willing to adopt new routines and to work around your disability; in short, be willing to live actively with your arthritis.

10. **Take responsibility.** It's not up to your doctor to "cure" you. Arthritis, more than most diseases, requires long-range planning and active participation on the part of the patient in order to realize the maximum benefit from treatment.

6.

FUTURE TREATMENTS

The future looks very bright for the treatment of arthritis. Researchers anticipate major break-throughs—not only in the treatment of arthritis symptoms but in the control of the fundamental disease processes that cause arthritis. There are two major reasons for this optimism.

First, many forms of arthritis result largely from a defect in the body's immume system. This de-fect in the immune system integrally connects ar-thritis research to the study of cancer, AIDS, and allergies—all conditions believed to be associated with the body's immune system. Therefore, the discoveries made as scientists learn more about these other diseases increase the chance of a ma-jor breakthrough for arthritis sufferers.

Second, because of the vast number of people afflicted with arthritis, there is a great financial inducement for the drug companies to discover a cure. The possibility of dominating the arthritis market is so powerful that it induces drug compa-nies to devote time and money to the research and development of potential breakthrough drugs.

Ironically, the drug companies' desire for such a new wonder drug should also make you very suspicious of news reports proclaiming an "amazing breakthrough in arthritis medication." The competition among drug companies is so intense that it may lead them to make misleading claims to physicians for their products. Always approach your medications with respect and caution—find out as much as you can about a medication before you take it, report any side effects to your doctor, and keep in close touch with him or her. And remember to be skeptical about "new" or "miracle" cures, even when they come from a seemingly trustworthy source.

Some of the breakthroughs in the next few years may involve the following treatments.

Immunoenhancing or Immunoregulatory Drugs

This is an experimental class of drugs that stimulate or enhance the body's immune response. Seemingly paradoxical, the theory is that in case the body's immune system may be reacting to a hidden agent, increasing rather than controlling the immune response may result in the agent's elimination, and therefore in improvement in the arthritic condition. These drugs are thought to be effective in some cases, but there are a great number of side effects, and, thus far, no indication for arthritis treatment is apparent.

13-cis-retinoic Acid

Researchers at Dartmouth-Hitchcock Medical Center have found this substance—a vitamin-A analogue—to significantly reduce joint inflammation in animals with experimentally induced arthritis.

Total Lymphoid Irradiation (TLI)

This is a technique, borrowed from cancer therapy, in which a radiation dose is administered over a period of five to six weeks to treat rheumatoid arthritis (RA). Experiments have been successful in significantly improving the condition of RA patients who have not responded to other treatments.

II

**The Most Commonly Prescribed
Arthritis Drugs in the
United States, Generic and Brand
Names, with Complete Descriptions
of Drugs and Their Effects**

1.

GENERAL INFORMATION ABOUT DRUG TYPES

Following is general information about the different types of drugs used to treat arthritis. Specific information about your drug can be found in the next section, where drugs are listed alphabetically by their generic names. If you have trouble locating any of your arthritis medications, please consult the index (see p. 193).

Analgesics

Aspirin (see p. 92)
Acetaminophen (see p. 88)

Aspirin is probably the closest thing we have to a wonder drug. It has been used for more than a century as a pain and fever remedy, but it is now used to treat a variety of conditions, including the inflammation associated with many forms of arthritis.

Aspirin is the anti-inflammatory against which

all other drugs of that class are compared. Chemically, aspirin is a member of the group of drugs called salicylates. Other salicylates are sodium salicylate, salsalate, sodium thiosalicylate, choline salicylate, and magnesium salicylate (all available in generic form). These drugs are no more effective than regular aspirin, although two of them (choline salicylate and magnesium salicylate) may be a little less irritating to the stomach. (This combination is marketed under the brand name Trilisate.) They are all more expensive than aspirin.

Interestingly, scientists believe they have finally learned how aspirin works. Its effects on pain and inflammation are thought to be related to its ability to prevent the manufacture of complex body hormones called prostaglandins. Of all the salicylates, aspirin has the greatest effect on prostaglandin production.

Many people find that they can take buffered aspirin but not regular aspirin. This is because in the buffered product, antacids have been added to the aspirin. The addition of the antacid is supposed to make the drug less irritating to the stomach and upper gastrointestinal tract. Otherwise, there is no difference between aspirin and buffered aspirin. The addition of antacids to aspirin may be important to people who must take large doses of aspirin for chronic arthritis or other conditions. In many cases, aspirin is the only effective drug.

Unlike aspirin, acetaminophen (Tylenol, Datril, etc.) does not inhibit prostaglandin production. Because it does not, acetaminophen reduces the chance of the user's suffering many of the side effects (such as an upset stomach) that may accompany aspirin.

Acetaminophen provides effective pain relief for a variety of conditions, including arthritic conditions involving musculoskeletal pain. However, acetaminophen is not recommended as an anti-inflammatory agent.

Both aspirin and acetaminophen are available in their less expensive generic forms.

In addition, many products contain acetaminophen and/or aspirin (or other salicylates) combined with other ingredients such as caffeine, antihistamines, barbiturates, meprobamate, and belladonna alkaloids. Caffeine is thought to help in the relief of pain associated with some forms of headaches; some popular products containing caffeine are Anacin, Excedrin, Midol, and Vanquish. Frequently, antihistamines, barbiturates, or meprobamate are provided for their sedative effects. Some of the products that contain these ingredients are Excedrin P.M. (contains an antihistamine and acetaminophen); Equagesic (aspirin and meprobamate); Fiorinal (aspirin, caffeine, and a barbiturate); and Bancap (acetaminophen and a barbiturate). Belladonna alkaloids, an ingredient in Dasin, are used to help settle the upset stomach that may accompany aspirin. All these products are often referred to as nonnarcotic pain relievers.

Nonsteroidal Anti-Inflammatory Drugs (NSAIDs)

Diflunisal (Dolobid)
Fenoprofen Calcium (see p. 116)
Ibuprofen (see p. 133)
Indomethacin (see p. 135)
Meclofenamate Sodium (see p. 139)
Mefenamic Acid (see p. 141)
Naproxen (and Naproxen Sodium) (see p. 147)
Oxyphenbutazone (see pg. 157)

Phenylbutazone (see pg. 157)
Piroxicam (see p. 165)
Sulindac (see p. 178)
Tolmetin Sodium (see p. 181)

Nonsteroidal anti-inflammatory drugs (NSAIDs) are a relatively new class of drugs used primarily to reduce the inflammation and pain caused by rheumatoid arthritis and osteoarthritis. Also, some NSAIDs are effective in acute gout and other inflammatory disorders of the musculoskeletal system, such as bursitis. These drugs are used for relief of acute pain in the long-term management of arthritis. NSAIDs do not stop the progression of arthritis. In general, NSAIDs are as effective as aspirin in relieving the signs and symptoms of arthritis, with fewer side effects. Many people who cannot tolerate aspirin may be able to take an NSAID. However, before taking an NSAID, it is important to inform your doctor of any side effects you may have incurred while taking aspirin. NSAIDs may be used with other antiarthritis medications such as corticosteroids and gold compounds. Using NSAIDs with aspirin is not recommended.

Corticosteroids

Betamethasone (see p. 97)
Cortisone (see p. 110)
Dexamethasone (see p. 113)
Fluprednisolone (see p. 119)
Hydrocortisone (see p. 127)
Methylprednisolone (see p. 144)
Paramethasone Acetate (see p. 160)
Prednisolone (see p. 168)
Prednisone (see p. 171)
Triamcinolone (see p. 184)

Corticosteroids are chemically related to naturally produced hormones that are essential to normal body functions. For this reason, these drugs may be prescribed for a wide variety of conditions ranging from skin rash to cancer. Corticosteroids are used in arthritis treatment because of their anti-inflammatory effects. The major differences among corticosteroids are the potency of medication and the variation in some secondary effects. Frequently, which corticosteroid you receive depends largely on your doctor's preference and past experience. These medications may be administered through injection, but most often are given in tablet form.

If you are on long-term corticosteroid therapy, you should wear or carry identification describing your medication.

Antigout Drugs

Allopurinol (see p. 90)
Colchicine (see p. 108)
Probenecid (see p. 174)
Sulfinpyrazone (see p. 176)

Probenecid and sulfinpyrazone are used to treat gout by increasing the body's urinary excretion of uric acid, thereby decreasing the level of uric acid in the blood. A high level of uric acid in the blood leads to the formation of crystals, which result in gouty arthritis.

Allopurinol reduces uric-acid levels by blocking the enzyme needed for the manufacture of uric acid in your body. A week or more of treatment may be needed before full effects of the drug are observed.

While no one knows exactly how colchicine works, it appears that it affects gout by reducing the body's inflammatory response to the crystals. Unlike drugs that affect uric-acid levels, colchicine will not block the progression of gout to chronic gouty arthritis, but it will relieve the pain of acute attacks and lessen the frequency and severity of attacks.

In addition to these drugs, indomethacin, naproxen, sulindac, phenylbutazone, and oxyphenbutazone are also indicated for the treatment of gout.

Gold Compounds

Gold Sodium Thioglucose (injection) (see p. 122)
Gold Sodium Thiomalate (injection) (see p. 124)
Auranofin (FDA approval pending)

Gold compounds are used to treat active rheumatoid arthritis and juvenile rheumatoid arthritis that have failed to respond to other conventional therapy such as aspirin and nonsteroidal anti-inflammatory drugs. Gold compounds are more effective if used in the early, active stages of arthritis, since it is believed they can suppress or prevent progression of the disease, but they cannot repair existing damage. The main drawback to gold treatment lies with the very high incidence of adverse effects: 25–50 percent of the patients report adverse effects while taking these drugs; 10 percent of the patients report serious toxic effects. Currently, gold compounds are available only through injection.

Auranofin (with the proposed brand name Ridaura) is an oral medication currently being investigated prior to approval by by the FDA. Many doctors look forward to its availability, since it appears that auranofin will have fewer side effects, while maintaining at least some of the benefits of injectable gold treatment.

Narcotic Pain Relievers

Codeine Phosphate with Acetaminophen (see p. 100)
Codeine Phosphate with Aspirin (see p. 104)
Codeine Sulfate with Aspirin (see p. 104)
Oxycodone Hydrochloride with Acetaminophen (see p. 150)
Oxycodone Hydrochloride with Aspirin (see p. 154)

These narcotic pain relievers may be prescribed to relieve the moderate to severe pain associated with many forms of arthritis. Because of the high abuse potential of these drugs, it is not recommended that they be taken for prolonged periods. Nonetheless, their use in relieving severe pain is of great value.

In recent decades, naturally occurring opium-based drugs have been largely replaced by a number of derivatives, or synthetics, that contain only a small amount of opium. The derivative drugs, like the originals, not only control pain; they can create a sense of intense euphoria, making them prime candidates for abuse.

Opium and opium-based drugs work by preventing pain signals from reaching the brain. Researchers have discovered that combining certain narcotics with nonprescription pain relievers like aspirin makes it possible to attain the same pain relief with lower doses of narcotics. These combination drugs have gained popularity within the medical community because the smaller narcotics dosage allows people to use the drug safely for longer periods of time.

Immunosuppressives

Azathioprine (see p. 96)

Immunosuppressives are used to inhibit the body's immune-response mechanism in the treatment of rheumatoid arthritis. It is recommended that azathioprine be used only by adult patients. Use of immunosuppressives should be restricted to *only* the severe, actively erosive form of rheumatoid arthritis that has not responded to more-conventional treatment such as aspirin, nonsteroidal drugs, or gold compounds.

In addition to treating rheumatoid arthritis, azathioprine is used in organ transplants to prevent the body's immune system from rejecting the transplanted organ. Currently, among immunosuppressives only azathioprine has been approved by the FDA for the treatment of rheumatoid arthritis. Other immunosuppressives, such as cyclophosphamide (Cytoxan), are being investigated for their potential use in arthritis treatment.

Penicillamine

Penicillamine (see p. 163)

No one knows exactly how penicillamine works in the treatment of rheumatoid arthritis, although it does seem to suppress the disease. Because penicillamine can cause severe adverse reactions, it should be used to treat only severe, active rheumatoid arthritis that has failed to respond to other treatment. It is also mandatory that, whenever possible, other treatment forms such as rest, physical therapy, salicylates (i.e., aspirin), and corticosteroids be used with penicillamine.

Penicillamine is a potent and potentially toxic drug with many *serious* side effects. Therefore, take this drug only under strict doctor's supervision and exactly as it is prescribed.

Antimalarial Drugs

Hydroxychloroquine Sulfate (see p. 131)

Hydroxychloroquine sulfate is an antimalarial drug that may be effective against moderate to severe rheumatoid arthritis and systemic lupus erythematosus, when these conditions have failed to respond to other therapy. In arthritis, hydroxychloroquine sulfate is used more often than other antimalarials (e.g., chloroquine) because it has fewer side effects; however, the long-term use of this drug may be limited by its potential toxic effects.

2.

DRUG PROFILES

Generic Name
Acetaminophen

Brand Names

A'Cenol	St. Joseph Aspirin-Free
Aceta	Sudoprin
Actamin	Tapanol Extra Strength
Anacin-3	Tapar
Banesin	Tempra
Conacetol	Tenol
Dapa	Tylenol
Datril Extra Strength	Ty-tabs
Febrigesic	Valadol
Febrinol	Valorin
Halenol Extra Strength	(Also available in generic
Panadol	form)
Panex	
Phenaphen	

Type of Drug

Analgesic

Prescribed for

Relief of mild to moderate pain associated with many forms of arthritis.

Cautions and Warnings

Do not take acetaminophen if you are allergic or sensitive to it.

Do not take acetaminophen for more than 10 days in a row unless directed to do so by your doctor. Do not exceed the recommended dosage.

Do not give acetaminophen to children under the age of 3 unless directed to do so by your doctor.

Use with caution if you suffer from liver disease. Consult your doctor immediately if pain persists for more than 10 days, if redness is present, or if a child under the age of 12 exhibits arthritic or rheumatic conditions.

Possible Side Effects

When used as directed, acetaminophen is relatively free of side effects. When side or adverse effects occur, they are usually the result of long-term use. Some of these side effects are: excitation, rash, and drowsiness.

Possible Adverse Effects

Associated with long-term use: jaundice (yellowing of the skin or whites of the eyes); fever; low blood sugar; disorders of the blood.

Drug Interactions

Oral contraceptives decrease the effectiveness of acetaminophen.

Activated charcoal, ingested immediately after acetaminophen, inhibits the absorption of acetaminophen.

Usual Dose

Adults: 300 to 650 mg. every 4 hours. Long-term therapy should not exceed 8 of the 325-mg. tablets daily.

Children:
Under 3 months: 40 mg.
4–11 months: 80 mg.
12–24 months: 120 mg.
2–3 years: 160 mg.
4–5 years: 240 mg.
6–8 years: 320 mg.
9–10 years: 400 mg.
11–12 years: 480 mg.

Children's doses may be repeated 4–5 times daily but should not exceed 5 doses. Do not give acetaminophen to children under the age of 3 unless directed to do so by your doctor.

Overdosage

Symptoms are bluish color of the lips, finger tips, etc.; rash; fever; stimulation; excitement; delirium; depression; nausea; vomiting; abdominal pain; diarrhea; yellowing of the skin and/or whites of the eyes; convulsions; coma. If you think you are experiencing an overdose, contact your doctor immediately, or go to a hospital emergency room. ALWAYS bring the medicine bottle with you.

Generic Name
Allopurinol

Brand Names

Lopurin
Zyloprim
(Also available in generic form)

ARTHRITIS

Drugs In Alphabetical Order

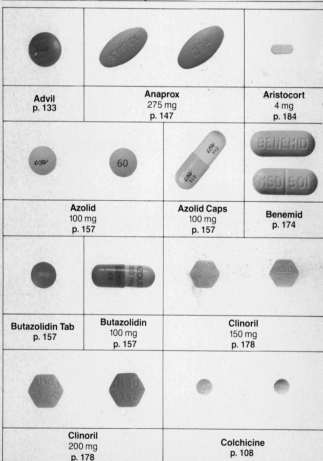

Advil
p. 133

Anaprox
275 mg
p. 147

Aristocort
4 mg
p. 184

Azolid
100 mg
p. 157

Azolid Caps
100 mg
p. 157

Benemid
p. 174

Butazolidin Tab
p. 157

Butazolidin
100 mg
p. 157

Clinoril
150 mg
p. 178

Clinoril
200 mg
p. 178

Colchicine
p. 108

A

Cortisone Acetate p. 110	Decadron .5 mg p. 113	Decadron .75 mg p. 113	Deltasone 5 mg p. 171
Deltasone 20 mg p. 171	Dexone 0.5 mg p. 113	Dexone 4 mg p. 113	Empirin Codeine 2 p. 104
Empirin Codeine 3 p. 104	Empirin Codeine 4 p. 104	Empracet #3 p. 101	Fiorinal Tab p. 104
Imuran 50 mg p. 96	Indocin 25 mg p. 135	Indocin 50 mg p. 135	Indocin SR 75 mg p. 135
Lopurin 100 mg p. 90	Meclomen 100 mg p. 139	Medrol Tabs 2 mg p. 144	

B

Medrol Tab 4 mg p. 144	**Meticorten** 1 mg p. 171	**Motrin** 300 mg p. 133
Motrin 400 mg p. 133	**Motrin** 600 mg p. 133	**Nalfon** 200 mg p. 116 **Nalfon** 300 mg p. 116
Nalfon 600 mg p. 116	**Naprosyn** 250 mg p. 147	
Naprosyn 375 mg p. 147	**Naprosyn** 500 mg p. 147	**Nuprin** 200 mg p. 133
Plaquenil p. 130	**Ponstel** 250 mg p. 141	**Prednisone** 10 mg p. 171

C

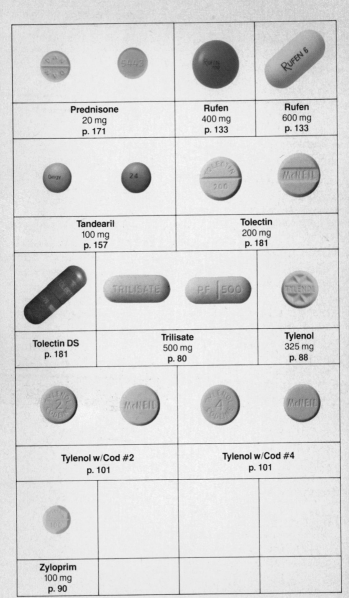

Prednisone 20 mg p. 171	**Rufen** 400 mg p. 133	**Rufen** 600 mg p. 133
Tandearil 100 mg p. 157	**Tolectin** 200 mg p. 181	
Tolectin DS p. 181	**Trilisate** 500 mg p. 80	**Tylenol** 325 mg p. 88
Tylenol w/Cod #2 p. 101	**Tylenol w/Cod #4** p. 101	
Zyloprim 100 mg p. 90		

D

Type of Drug

Reduces the production of uric acid

Prescribed for

Gouty arthritis.

Cautions and Warnings

Do not take allopurinol if you have ever developed a severe reaction to it in the past.

Notify your doctor immediately if you develop a skin rash.

Children should not use allopurinol, except when their high uric-acid levels are due to a malignancy.

Mothers should not breast-feed while using allopurinol, since it will pass through mother's milk into the child.

Pregnant women should use this drug only when the benefits clearly outweigh the unknown potential hazards to the fetus.

Allopurinol can make you sleepy; therefore, use caution while driving or performing tasks that require concentration.

It is important that you drink 10 to 12 glasses (8 ounces each glass) of water each day.

Use allopurinol with extreme caution if you suffer from kidney or liver disease. It may be necessary for you to undergo liver-function tests, especially in the early stages of allopurinol therapy.

To prevent upset stomach, take allopurinol with food.

Possible Side Effects

Skin rash; nausea; vomiting; diarrhea; drowsiness; intermittent stomach pains; itching.

Possible Adverse Effects

Fever; chills; loss of hair; effects on blood components; lack of concentration; rarely, effects on the eyes.

Drug Interactions

Large doses of vitamin C may increase the possibility of kidney-stone formation.

Possible interaction with drugs to treat cancer is important and should be taken into account by your doctor.

Allopurinol may prolong the life of anticoagulant (blood-thinning) medication such as dicumarol. Therefore, your doctor may have to adjust your dosage of anticoagulants if you are taking allopurinol.

Usual Dose

100 to 300 mg. daily depending on the severity of the disease and your response to the medication.

Overdosage

There have been no reports of a massive overdose with allopurinol. However, if you think you are experiencing an overdose reaction, call your doctor immediately, or go to a hospital emergency room. ALWAYS bring the medicine bottle with you.

Generic Name
Aspirin

Brand Names

A.S.A.
Arthritis Bayer

Buffered Aspirin
Arthritis Pain Formula

Buffered Aspirin (cont.)

Bayer	Ascriptin
Bayer Children's	Asperbuf
Cospirin	Buff-A
Easpirin	Buffaprin
Ecotrin	Bufferin
Empirin	Buffex
Hipirin	Buffinol
Measurin	Buf-Tabs
Norwich Aspirin	Cama Arthritis Strength
St. Joseph Aspirin for	Wesprin Buffered
Children	
Zorprin	

(Also available in generic form)

Type of Drug

Analgesic and anti-inflammatory

Prescribed for

Relief of mild to moderate pain, and reduction of inflammation associated with rheumatoid arthritis, juvenile rheumatoid arthritis, and osteoarthritis.

Cautions and Warnings

Do not use aspirin if you are allergic to any other salicylate, to nonsteroidal anti-inflammatory drugs (NSAIDs)—e.g., indomethacin, ibuprofen, naproxen, etc. The most common allergic reaction to aspirin involves asthmalike symptoms within 3 hours of taking aspirin. People who have asthma and/or nasal polyps are more likely to be allergic to aspirin.

The use of salicylates, especially aspirin, in children with flu or chickenpox may be associated with the development of a very rare but potentially fatal condition called Reye's syndrome. While the role of aspirin in the development of Reye's syndrome is not clear, the Surgeon General of the United States recommends that children with flu or chickenpox NOT be given any salicylates (including aspirin).

Do not use aspirin if you suffer from hemophilia, bleeding ulcers, or any hemorrhaging conditions, or if you suffer from severe kidney or liver disease.

Do not use aspirin if you are pregnant, since it may produce adverse effects in both the mother and the fetus.

Avoid aspirin if you are allergic to tartrazine.

Notify your doctor if ringing in the ears occurs, or if you experience persistent upset stomach.

Do not use aspirin if it has a strong vinegarlike smell (this odor means that aspirin effectiveness has expired).

To minimize stomach upset, take aspirin with food or milk.

Possible Side Effects

Heartburn; loss of appetite; upset stomach; nausea; small amounts of blood in the stool.

Possible Adverse Effects

Hives; rash; runny nose; asthmalike symptoms; gastrointestinal bleeding; ulcers.

Drug Interactions

People taking anticoagulants (blood thinners) should avoid aspirin. The effect of the anticoagulant will be increased.

The risks of ulcers occurring is increased when aspirin is taken with steroids, phenylbutazone, or alcohol.

Aspirin decreases the effects of probenecid, sulfinpyrazone, and furosemide.

Propranolol may decrease aspirin's anti-inflammatory effects.

Phenobarbital decreases the effects of aspirin.

Aspirin may increase the glucose-lowering effects of sulfonylureas and insulin.

Usual Dose

Minor aches and pains: 325 to 650 mg. every 4 hours if necessary.

Arthritis and rheumatic conditions: 2.6 to 5.2 grams per day in divided doses.

Juvenile rheumatoid arthritis: 90 to 130 mg. per 2.2 lbs. of body weight every 24 hours in 4- to 6-hour intervals.

Overdosage

Mild overdosage: rapid and deep breathing; nausea; vomiting; dizziness; ringing or buzzing in the ears; flushing; sweating; thirst; headache; drowsiness; diarrhea; rapid heartbeat.

Symptoms of severe overdosage: fever; excitement; confusion; convulsions; coma; excessive bleeding.

The initial treatment of aspirin overdosage involves making the patient vomit to remove any aspirin remaining in the stomach. DO NOT IN-DUCE VOMITING UNTIL YOU HAVE SPOKEN WITH YOUR DOCTOR OR POISON-CONTROL CENTER. If in doubt, go to a hospital emergency room. AL-WAYS bring the medicine bottle with you.

Generic Name
Azathioprine

Brand Name

Imuran

Type of Drug

Immunosuppressive

Prescribed for

Rheumatoid arthritis.

Cautions and Warnings

Whenever possible, pregnant women should not use azathioprine.

Notify your doctor if you experience unusual bleeding or bruising; fever; sore throat; mouth sores; any signs of infection; stomach pain; pale stools; darkened urine.

Also notify your doctor if you suffer persistent or bothersome nausea; vomiting; skin rash; aches; pains; diarrhea.

To prevent upset stomach, take azathioprine with food.

Azathioprine can cause cancer in animals, and there is a risk that its use may lead to cancer in humans. It is mandatory that you remain under your doctor's care while taking azathioprine.

Possible Side Effects

The most often seen and most severe side effects are related to the blood. These may manifest themselves by unusual bleeding or be detected by weekly blood counts.

Possible Adverse Effects

Mouth sores; fever; loss of hair; joint pains; nausea; vomiting; diarrhea; loss of appetite; yellowing of the skin and/or whites of the eyes.

Drug Interactions

Allopurinol reduces the rate at which azathioprine is eliminated from the body. This interaction may result in the need to lower your azathioprine dose to ⅓ or ¼ of its normal level.

The combined use of azathioprine with gold, antimalarials, or penicillamine has not been evaluated and therefore cannot be recommended.

Usual Dose

50 to 100 mg. daily. This dosage may be increased after 6 to 8 weeks up to a maximum dose of 125 to 250 mg.

Generic Name
Betamethasone

Brand Name

Celestone

Type of Drug

Corticosteroid

Prescribed for

Rheumatoid arthritis; osteoarthritis; ankylosing

spondylitis; acute gout; juvenile rheumatoid arthritis; psoriasis; systemic lupus erythematosus; polymyositis; many other nonarthritic conditions.

Cautions and Warnings

Avoid abrupt withdrawal of betamethasone. Notify your doctor if, after having your dosage reduced or stopped, you experience fatigue; loss of appetite; weight loss; nausea; vomiting; diarrhea; weakness; dizziness.

Take betamethasone with food to avoid upset stomach. Single daily doses, or every-other-day doses, should be taken preferably before 9:00 A.M. Multiple doses should be spread out evenly throughout the day.

Notify your doctor if you experience unusual weight gain; swelling of the ankles or feet; weakness; black tarry stools; vomiting of blood; heartburn; facial puffiness; menstrual irregularities; prolonged sore throat; fever; cold; infection. (Since betamethasone may mask symptoms of infection, it is very important that you report anything that you suspect may be an infection.)

If you are taking betamethasone, you should not be vaccinated against infectious diseases.

Pregnant women, women of childbearing potential, and nursing mothers should use betamethasone only when the potential benefits clearly outweigh the unknown potential hazards to the fetus. If you become pregnant while taking betamethasone, please notify your doctor.

Very stressful situations (such as an accident) may require an increase in dosage.

If you are on long-term betamethasone therapy, you should wear or carry identification describing your medication.

If you are sensitive to aspirin or tartrazine, you may be allergic to betamethasone.

Use with caution if you suffer from high blood pressure or kidney, liver, thyroid, or heart disease.

Your doctor may prescribe a calcium supplement to help prevent osteoporosis.

Possible Side Effects

Upset stomach; water retention; heart failure; potassium loss; muscle weakness; loss of muscle mass; calcium loss (osteoporosis); slow healing from wounds; black and blue marks; sweating; itching; rash; dizziness; headache.

Possible Adverse Effects

Slowing down of growth in children; depression of the adrenal and/or pituitary glands; diabetes; glaucoma; hypersensitivity or allergic reactions; blood clots; insomnia; weight gain; increased appetite; nausea; feeling of ill health. Psychic derangements may appear, ranging from euphoria to mood swings, personality changes, insomnia, and severe depression.

Drug Interactions

If you are diabetic, betamethasone may cause the need for an increase in your antidiabetic medication.

Phenytoin, phenobarbital, rifampin, and possibly ephedrine may cause the need for an alteration in your betamethasone dosage.

Betamethasone may affect anticoagulant dosages.

Drugs that reduce serum-cholesterol levels, such as cholestyramine and colestipol, may decrease the effects of betamethasone.

Interaction with diuretics may cause you to lose potassium. Be aware of signs of lowered potassium levels, such as weakness, muscle cramps, and tiredness, and report them to your doctor. Your doctor may recommend that you take a potassium supplement, or that you eat foods rich in potassium, such as bananas, citrus fruits, melon, and tomatoes.

Use aspirin with caution while taking betamethasone.

Usual Dose

Initial dose: 0.6 to 7.2 mg. daily. Then adjusted to suit your needs.

Overdosage

Overdosage of betamethasone may result in anxiety; depression; confusion; high blood pressure; elevated blood sugar; stomach cramps or bleeding; swelling of the hands or feet; purplish skin patches. If you experience any of these symptoms, contact your doctor immediately, or go to a hospital emergency room. ALWAYS bring the medicine bottle with you.

Generic Name
Codeine Phosphate with Acetaminophen

Brand Names

Aceta with Codeine
Amaphen with Codeine
Anacin-3 with Codeine
Bancap with Codeine

Capital with Codeine
Codalan
Codap
Empracet with Codeine
G-2; G-3
Maxigesic
Panadol with Codeine
Phenaphen with Codeine
Proval No. 3
Tega-Code-M
Tylenol with Codeine
Ty-Tab
(Also available generically as acetaminophen with codeine)

Type of Drug

Narcotic pain reliever combined with nonprescription pain reliever

Prescribed for

Relief of mild to moderate pain.

Cautions and Warnings

Do not take codeine phosphate with acetaminophen if you know you are allergic or sensitive to it. Use this drug with extreme caution if you suffer from asthma or other breathing problems. Long-term use of codeine phosphate with acetaminophen may cause drug dependence or addiction. Codeine is a respiratory depressant and affects the central nervous system, producing sleepiness, tiredness, and/or inability to concentrate. Be careful if you are driving, operating machinery, or performing other functions that require concentration. If you are pregnant or suspect that you are pregnant, do not take this drug.

Codeine phosphate with acetaminophen is best taken with food to prevent stomach upset.

Possible Side Effects

Most frequent: light-headedness; dizziness; sleepiness; nausea; vomiting; loss of appetite; sweating. If these occur, ask your doctor about lowering your dose of codeine phosphate with acetaminophen. Usually the side effects disappear if you simply lie down.

If you experience shallow breathing or difficulty in breathing, call your doctor immediately or go to the hospital.

Possible Adverse Effects

Euphoria (feeling high); weakness; sleepiness; headache; agitation; uncoordinated muscle movement; minor hallucinations; disorientation and visual disturbances; dry mouth; loss of appetite; constipation; flushing of the face; rapid heartbeat; palpitations; faintness; urinary difficulties or hesitancy; reduced sex drive and/or potency; itching; rash; anemia; lowered blood sugar; yellowing of the skin and/or whites of the eyes. Narcotic pain relievers may aggravate convulsions in those who have had convulsions in the past.

Drug Interactions

Because of its depressant effect and potential effect on breathing, codeine phosphate with acetaminophen should be taken with extreme care in combination with alcohol, sleeping medicine, tranquilizers, or other depressant drugs.

Dependence and Addiction

Most people are aware that narcotics have an extremely high potential for abuse and addiction. This varies according to the strength of the particular drug, frequency of use, the circumstances under which it is used, and the individual's susceptibility to addiction.

It is very important that you inform your doctor about any problems that you or any member of your family has had with alcohol or tranquilizers.

Dependence to narcotics manifests itself through increased tolerance to the drug's pain relief; if you notice that the pain won't go away unless you increase your dosage, you may be becoming dependent on the narcotic.

The major signs of addiction include varying degrees of anxiety when the drug is suddenly withdrawn.

Withdrawal Symptoms

Yawning; excessive sweating; sneezing; twitching and kicking; tremors; gooseflesh; fever and chills alternating with flushing; anxiety; dilated pupils; over-all weakness and aches; loss of appetite; nausea; vomiting; diarrhea; cramps.

Withdrawal Treatment

Treatment for narcotic withdrawal, which should be handled *only* by trained medical personnel, often includes the use of sedatives to ease anxiety, after which the narcotic is gradually withdrawn over a period of several days.

Usual Dose

Adults: 1 to 2 tablets every 4 hours.
Children: Not recommended for children.

Overdosage

Symptoms are depression of respiration (breathing); extreme tiredness progressing to stupor and then coma; pinpointed pupils of the eyes; no response to stimulation such as a pinprick; cold and clammy skin; slowing of the heart rate; lowering of blood pressure; yellowing of the skin and/or whites of the eyes; bluish color in skin of hands and feet; fever; excitement; delirium; convulsions; cardiac arrest; liver toxicity (shown by nausea, vomiting, pain in the abdomen, and diarrhea). If you think you are experiencing an overdose, go to a hospital emergency room immediately. ALWAYS bring the medicine bottle with you.

Generic Names

Codeine Phosphate with Aspirin
Codeine Sulfate with Aspirin

Brand Names

Anexsia with Codeine
A.S.A. & Codeine Compound
Ascriptin with Codeine
Buff-A Comp
Bufferin with Codeine
Emcodeine Tablets
Empirin with Codeine
Fiorinal with Codeine

Type of Drug

Narcotic pain reliever combined with nonprescription pain reliever

Prescribed for

Relief of mild to moderate pain.

Cautions and Warnings

Do not take this drug if you know you are allergic or sensitive to it. Use codeine phosphate with aspirin (or codeine sulfate with aspirin) with extreme caution if you suffer from asthma or other breathing problems. Long-term use of this drug may cause drug dependence or addiction. Codeine is a respiratory depressant and affects the central nervous system, producing sleepiness, tiredness, and/or inability to concentrate. If you are pregnant or suspect that you are pregnant, do not take this drug.

Drowsiness may occur: be careful when driving or operating hazardous machinery.

Codeine phosphate with aspirin (or codeine sulfate with aspirin) is best taken with food to prevent stomach upset.

Possible Side Effects

Most frequent: light-headedness; dizziness; sleepiness; nausea; vomiting; loss of appetite; sweating. If these occur, ask your doctor about lowering your dose of codeine. Usually the side effects disappear if you simply lie down.

If you experience shallow breathing or difficulty in breathing, call your doctor immediately, or go to the hospital.

Possible Adverse Effects

Euphoria (feeling high); weakness; sleepiness; headache; agitation; uncoordinated muscle movement; minor hallucinations; disorientation and visual disturbances; dry mouth; loss of appetite; constipation; flushing of the face; rapid heartbeat; palpitations; faintness; urinary difficulties or hesitancy; reduced sex drive and/or potency; itching; rash; anemia; lowered blood sugar; yellowing of the skin and/or whites of the eyes. Narcotic pain relievers may aggravate convulsions in those who have had convulsions in the past.

Drug Interactions

Interaction with alcohol, tranquilizers, barbiturates, or sleeping pills produces tiredness, sleepiness, or inability to concentrate, and seriously increases the depressive effect of this drug.

The aspirin ingredient can affect anticoagulant (blood-thinning) therapy. Be sure to discuss this with your doctor so that the proper dosage adjustment can be made.

Interaction with corticosteriods, phenylbutazone, or alcohol can cause severe stomach irritation with possible bleeding.

Dependence and Addiction

Most people are aware that narcotics have an extremely high potential for abuse and addiction. This varies according to the strength of the particular drug, frequency of use, the circumstances under which it is used, and the individual's susceptibility to addiction.

It is very important that you inform your doctor about any problems that you or any member of your family has had with alcohol or tranquilizers.

Dependence to narcotics manifests itself through increased tolerance to drug's pain relief; if you notice that the pain won't go away unless you increase your dosage, you may be becoming dependent on the narcotic.

The major signs of addiction include varying degrees of anxiety when the drug is suddenly withdrawn.

Withdrawal Symptoms

Yawning; excessive sweating; sneezing; twitching and kicking; tremors; gooseflesh; fever and chills alternating with flushing; anxiety; dilated pupils; over-all weakness and aches; loss of appetite; nausea; vomiting; diarrhea; cramps.

Withdrawal Treatment

Treatment for narcotic withdrawal, which should be handled *only* by trained medical personnel, often includes the use of sedatives to ease anxiety, after which the narcotic is gradually withdrawn over a period of several days.

Usual Dose

Adults: 1 to 2 tablets 3 to 4 times per day.
Children: Not recommended for children.

Overdosage

Symptoms are depression of respiration (breathing); extreme tiredness progressing to stupor and then coma; pinpointed pupils of the eyes; no response to stimulation such as a pinprick; cold and clammy skin; slowing of the heartbeat; lowering of blood pressure; convulsions; cardiac arrest. If you think you are experiencing an overdose, go to a hospital emergency room immediately. ALWAYS bring the medicine bottle with you.

Generic Name
Colchicine

Brand Name

Colsalide
(Also available in generic form)

Type of Drug

Reduces the inflammatory response to gout crystals

Prescribed for

Gouty arthritis.

Cautions and Warnings

Notify your doctor if you experience skin rash; sore throat; fever; unusual bleeding or bruising; tiredness; numbness; tingling.

Stop taking colchicine as soon as gout pain is relieved or at the first sign of nausea, vomiting, stomach pain, or diarrhea. If you experience these side effects, contact your doctor.

Do not use colchicine if you suffer from serious kidney, liver, stomach, or cardiac disorder.

Colchicine should be used with great caution by the elderly.

Colchicine can harm the fetus; use by pregnant women should be considered only when the benefits clearly outweigh the potential hazards to the fetus.

Safety and effectiveness for use by children has not been established.

Periodic blood counts should be done when you are taking colchicine for long periods of time.

Possible Side Effects

Vomiting; diarrhea; stomach pain; nausea; hair loss; skin rash.

Possible Adverse Effects

Disorders of the blood may occur in patients undergoing long-term colchicine therapy.

Drug Interactions

Colchicine has been shown to cause poor absorption of vitamin B-12, a condition that is reversible.

Colchicine may increase sensitivity to central-nervous-system depressants such as tranquilizers and alcohol.

Usual Dose

To relieve an acute attack of gout: 1 to 1.2 mg. This dose may be followed by 0.5 to 1.2 mg. every 1 to 2 hours until pain is relieved. The total amount usually needed to control pain and inflammation during an attack varies from 4 to 8 mg.

To prevent gout attacks: 0.3 to 1.2 mg. daily.

Overdose

Symptoms of colchicine overdose may include: nausea; vomiting; stomach pain; burning sensations in the throat, stomach, and skin; diarrhea (which may be severe and bloody). If you think you are experiencing an overdose, contact your doctor immediately, or go to a hospital emergency room. ALWAYS bring the medicine bottle with you.

Generic Name

Cortisone Acetate

Brand Name

Cortone Acetate
(Also available in generic form)

Type of Drug

Corticosteroid

Prescribed for

Rheumatoid arthritis; osteoarthritis; ankylosing spondylitis; acute gout; juvenile rheumatoid arthritis; psoriasis; systemic lupus erythematosus; polymyositis; many other nonarthritic conditions.

Cautions and Warnings

Avoid abrupt withdrawal of cortisone. Notify your doctor if, after having your dosage reduced or stopped, you experience fatigue; loss of appetite; weight loss; nausea; vomiting; diarrhea; weakness; dizziness.

Take cortisone with food to avoid upset stomach. Single daily doses, or every-other-day doses, should be taken perferably before 9:00 A.M. Multiple doses should be spread out evenly throughout the day.

Notify your doctor if you experience unusual weight gain; swelling of the ankles or feet; weakness; black tarry stools; vomiting of blood; heartburn; facial puffiness; menstrual irregularities; prolonged sore throat; fever; cold; infection. (Since cortisone may mask symptoms of infection, it is very important that you report anything that you suspect may be an infection.)

If you are taking cortisone you should not be vaccinated against infectious diseases.

Pregnant women, women of childbearing potential, and nursing mothers should use cortisone only when the potential benefits clearly outweigh the unknown potential hazards to the fetus. If you become pregnant while taking cortisone, please notify your doctor.

Very stressful situations (such as an accident) may require an increase in dosage.

If you are on long-term cortisone therapy, you should wear or carry identification describing your medication.

If you are sensitive to aspirin or tartrazine, you may be allergic to cortisone.

Use with caution if you suffer from high blood pressure or kidney, liver, thyroid, or heart disease.

Your doctor may prescribe a calcium supplement to help prevent osteoporosis.

Possible Side Effects

Upset stomach; water retention; heart failure; potassium loss; muscle weakness; loss of muscle mass; calcium loss (osteoporosis); slow healing from wounds; black and blue marks; sweating; itching; rash; dizziness; headache.

Possible Adverse Effects

Slowing down of growth in children; depression of the adrenal and/or pituitary glands; diabetes; glaucoma; hypersensitivity or allergic reactions; blood clots; insomnia; weight gain; increased appetite; nausea; feeling of ill health. Psychic derangements may appear, ranging from euphoria to mood swings, personality changes, insomnia, and severe depression.

Drug Interactions

If you are diabetic, cortisone may cause the need for an increase in your antidiabetic medication.

Phenytoin, phenobarbital, rifampin, and possibly ephedrine may cause the need for an alteration in your cortisone dosage.

Cortisone may affect anticoagulant dosages.

Drugs that reduce serum-cholesterol levels, such as cholestyramine and colestipol, may decrease the effects of cortisone.

Interaction with diuretics may cause you to lose potassium. Be aware of signs of lowered potassium levels, such as weakness, muscle cramps, and tiredness, and report them to your doctor. Your doctor may recommend that you take a potassium supplement, or that you eat foods rich in potassium, such as bananas, citrus fruits, melon, and tomatoes.

Use aspirin with caution while taking cortisone.

Usual Dose

Initial dose: 20 to 300 mg. daily. Then adjusted to suit your needs.

Overdosage

Overdosage of cortisone may result in anxiety; depression; confusion; high blood pressure; elevated blood sugar; stomach cramps or bleeding; swelling of the hands or feet; purplish skin patches. If you experience any of these symptoms, contact your doctor immediately, or go to a hospital emergency room. ALWAYS bring the medicine bottle with you.

Generic Name
Dexamethasone

Brand Names

Decadron
Dexameth
Dexone
Hexadrol
(Also available in generic form)

Type of Drug

Corticosteroid

Prescribed for

Rheumatoid arthritis; osteoarthritis; ankylosing spondylitis; acute gout; juvenile rheumatoid arthritis; psoriasis; systemic lupus erythematosus; polymyositis; many other nonarthritic conditions.

Cautions and Warnings

Avoid abrupt withdrawal of dexamethasone. Notify your doctor if, after having your dosage reduced or stopped, you experience fatigue; loss of appetite; weight loss; nausea; vomiting; diarrhea; weakness; dizziness.

Take dexamethasone with food to avoid upset stomach. Single daily doses, or every-other-day doses, should be taken preferably before 9:00 A.M. Multiple doses should be spread out evenly throughout the day.

Notify your doctor if you experience unusual weight gain; swelling of the ankles or feet; weakness; black tarry stools; vomiting of blood; heartburn; facial puffiness; menstrual irregularities; prolonged sore throat; fever; cold; infection. (Since dexamethasone may mask symptoms of infection, it is very important that you report anything that you suspect may be an infection.)

If you are taking dexamethasone, you should not be vaccinated against infectious diseases.

Pregnant women, women of childbearing potential, and nursing mothers should use dexamethasone only when the potential benefits clearly outweigh the unknown potential hazards to the fetus. If you become pregnant while taking dexamethasone, please notify your doctor.

Very stressful situations (such as an accident) may require an increase in dosage.

If you are on long-term dexamethasone therapy, you should wear or carry identification describing your medication.

If you are sensitive to aspirin or tartrazine, you may be allergic to dexamethasone.

Use with caution if you suffer from high blood pressure or kidney, liver, thyroid, or heart disease.

Your doctor may prescribe a calicum supplement to help prevent osteoporosis.

Possible Side Effects

Upset stomach; water retention; heart failure; potassium loss; muscle weakness; loss of muscle mass; calcium loss (osteoporosis); slow healing from wounds; black and blue marks; sweating; itching; rash; dizziness; headache.

Possible Adverse Effects

Slowing down of growth in children; depression of the adrenal and/or pituitary glands; diabetes; glaucoma; hypersensitivity or allergic reactions; blood clots; insomnia; weight gain; increased appetite; nausea; feeling of ill health. Psychic derangements may appear, ranging from euphoria to mood swings, personality changes, insomnia, and severe depression.

Drug Interactions

If you are diabetic, dexamethasone may cause the need for an increase in your antidiabetic medication.

Phenytoin, phenobarbital, rifampin, and possibly ephedrine may cause the need for an alteration in your dexamethasone dosage.

Dexamethasone may affect anticoagulant dosages.

Drugs that reduce serum-cholesterol levels, such as cholestyramine and colestipol, may decrease the effects of dexamethasone.

Interaction with diuretics may cause you to lose potassium. Be aware of signs of lowered potassium levels, such as weakness, muscle cramps, and tiredness, and report them to your doctor. Your doctor may recommend that you take a potassium supplement or that you eat foods rich in potassium, such as bananas, citrus fruits, melon, and tomatoes.

Use aspirin with caution while taking dexamethasone.

Usual Dose

Initial dose: 0.75 to 9 mg. daily. Then adjusted to suit your needs.

Overdosage

Overdosage of dexamethasone may result in anxiety; depression; confusion; high blood pressure; elevated blood sugar; stomach cramps or bleeding; swelling of the hands or feet; purplish skin patches. If you experience any of these symptoms, contact your doctor immediately, or go to a hospital emergency room. ALWAYS bring the medicine bottle with you.

Generic Name
Fenoprofen Calcium

Brand Name

Nalfon

Type of Drug

Nonsteroidal anti-inflammatory

Prescribed for

Rheumatoid arthritis, osteoarthritis, relief of mild to moderate pain.

Cautions and Warnings

Do not use fenoprofen calcium if you have had an allergic reaction to aspirin or any other nonsteroidal anti-inflammatory drug (NSAID).

Use with caution if you have a history of kidney, liver, or heart disease; high blood pressure; defects in the blood's clotting ability; or are currently taking anticoagulant medication. If you are suffering from an active peptic ulcer, it is recommended that other forms of drug therapy be tried before using fenoprofen calcium.

With elderly patients, it is recommended that reduced dosages be instituted initially.

Use by pregnant women or nursing mothers is not recommended.

Anemia may occur in patients undergoing long-term therapy with fenoprofen calcium. If you are anemic, is suggested that you have your hemoglobin values determined frequently.

Pay special attention to any changes in your vision (blurred or partially obstructed vision or color blindness) or any eye complaints that occur when taking fenoprofen calcium. Blurred vision is especially significant and requires a thorough eye examination. It is also recommended that you have your eyes checked regularly if you are undergoing prolonged therapy with fenoprofen calcium.

Avoid aspirin while taking fenoprofen calcium.

Fenoprofen calcium may cause dizziness, drowsiness, or blurred vision; therefore, use caution while driving or performing tasks that require concentration.

Do not use fenoprofen calcium if you have a history of seriously impaired kidney function.

The safety of using fenoprofen calcium in patients who have impaired hearing has not been proved; it is suggested that periodic hearing tests be performed during long-term therapy with fenoprofen calcium.

To minimize upset stomach, take fenoprofen calcium with food.

Possible Side Effects

Nausea; vomiting; diarrhea; constipation; upset stomach; dizziness; headache; drowsiness; nervousness; insomnia; asthma; heartburn; anemia.

Possible Adverse Effects

Irregular heartbeat; low blood pressure; chest

pain; swelling of the hands or feet; adverse effects on the blood; unusual bleeding.

Drug Interactions

Using fenoprofen calcium while taking anticoagulants may require a reduction of anticoagulant medication.

Aspirin may decrease the effectiveness of fenoprofen calcium and probably should not be combined.

Probenecid may enhance the effects of fenoprofen calcium; therefore, a reduced fenoprofen calcium dosage may be necessary when taking probenecid.

Fenoprofen calcium may increase the effects of anticonvulsants, antidiabetics, and sulfa drugs; your doctor may change the dosages of these other drugs.

Avoid alcohol, since this may increase stomach irritation and drowsiness.

Usual Dose

Rheumatoid and osteoarthritis: 300 to 600 mg. 3 or 4 times daily. It may take 2 or 3 weeks before the benefits of drug therapy are noticed.

Mild to moderate pain relief: 200 mg. every 4 to 6 hours, as necessary.

Do not exceed 3,200 mg. daily.

Safety and effectiveness for children has not been established.

Overdosage

In general, NSAID overdosage is treated by inducing vomiting, followed by the administration of activated charcoal. *However, do NOT induce vomiting or use activated charcoal unless directed to do so by your doctor or poison-control center.* When in doubt, proceed to a hospital emergency room. ALWAYS bring the medicine bottle with you.

Generic Name
Fluprednisolone

Brand Name

Alphadrol

Type of Drug

Corticosteroid

Prescribed for

Rheumatoid arthritis; osteoarthritis; ankylosing spondylitis; acute gout; juvenile rheumatoid arthritis; psoriasis; systemic lupus erythematosus; polymyositis; many other nonarthritic conditions.

Cautions and Warnings

Avoid abrupt withdrawal of fluprednisolone. Notify your doctor if, after having your dosage reduced or stopped, you experience fatigue; loss of appetite; weight loss; nausea; vomiting; diarrhea; weakness; dizziness.

Take fluprednisolone with food to avoid upset stomach. Single daily doses, or every-other-day doses, should be taken preferably before 9:00 A.M. Multiple doses should be spread out evenly throughout the day.

Notify your doctor if you experience unusual weight gain; swelling of the ankles or feet; weakness; black tarry stools; vomiting of blood; heartburn; facial puffiness; menstrual irregularities; prolonged sore throat; fever; cold; infection. (Since fluprednisolone may mask symptoms of infection, it is very important that you report anything that you suspect may be an infection.)

If you are taking fluprednisolone, you should not be vaccinated against infectious diseases.

Pregnant women, women of childbearing potential, and nursing mothers should use fluprednisolone only when the potential benefits clearly outweigh the unknown potential hazards to the fetus. If you become pregnant while taking fluprednisolone, please notify your doctor.

Very stressful situations (such as an accident) may require an increase in dosage.

If you are on long-term fluprednisolone therapy, you should wear or carry identification describing your medication.

If you are sensitive to aspirin or tartrazine, you may be allergic to fluprednisolone.

Use with caution if you suffer from high blood pressure or kidney, liver, thyroid, or heart disease.

Your doctor may prescribe a calcium supplement to help prevent osteoporosis.

Possible Side Effects

Upset stomach; water retention; heart failure; potassium loss; muscle weakness; loss of muscle mass; calcium loss (osteoporosis); slow healing from wounds; black and blue marks; sweating; itching; rash; dizziness; headache.

Possible Adverse Effects

Slowing down of growth in children; depression of the adrenal and/or pituitary glands; diabetes; glaucoma; hypersensitivity or allergic reactions;

blood clots; insomnia; weight gain; increased appetite; nausea; feeling of ill health. Psychic derangements may appear, ranging from euphoria to mood swings, personality changes, insomnia, and severe depression.

Drug Interactions

If you are diabetic, fluprednisolone may cause the need for an increase in your antidiabetic medication.

Phenytoin, phenobarbital, rifampin, and possibly ephedrine may cause the need for an alteration in your fluprednisolone dosage.

Fluprednisolone may affect anticoagulant dosages.

Drugs that reduce serum-cholesterol levels, such as cholestyramine and colestipol, may decrease the effects of fluprednisolone.

Interaction with diuretics may cause you to lose potassium. Be aware of signs of lowered potassium levels, such as weakness, muscle cramps, and tiredness, and report them to your doctor. Your doctor may recommend that you eat foods rich in potassium, such as bananas, citrus fruits, melon, and tomatoes.

Use aspirin with caution while taking fluprednisolone.

Usual Dose

Initial dosage: 2.5 to 30 mg. daily. Then adjusted to suit your needs.

Overdosage

Overdosage of fluprednisolone may result in anxiety; depression; confusion; high blood pressure; elevated blood sugar; stomach cramps or bleeding; swelling of the hands or feet; purplish skin patches. If you experience any of these symptoms, contact your doctor immediately, or go to a hospital emergency room. ALWAYS bring the medicine bottle with you.

Generic Name
Gold Sodium Thioglucose

Brand Name

Solganal

Type of Drug

Gold compound

Prescribed for

Rheumatoid arthritis and juvenile rheumatoid arthritis.

Cautions and Warnings

Do not use aurothioglucose if you have uncontrolled diabetes; kidney or liver disease; a history of infectious hepatitis; marked high blood pressure; heart failure; systemic lupus erythematosus; abnormal blood cells; recently been exposed to radiation; had a severe toxic reaction previously to gold therapy; hives; eczema; colitis; or if you are in a severely debilitated state characterized by very poor circulation to the brain or body.

Notify your doctor if you experience skin rash; loss of hair or nails; inflammation of the mouth; mouth ulcers; metallic taste in the mouth; fever;

cough; shortness of breath; fainting; slow heart-beat; thickening of the tongue; difficulty in swallowing and breathing; swelling of the eyelids or lips; nausea; vomiting; stomach cramps; diarrhea; loss of appetite; severe stomach pain. Some of these reactions may be very serious, so it is important that you contact your doctor promptly if you experience any of them.

Skin discoloration and rashes may occur as a result of exposure to sunlight. In addition, careful oral hygiene is important.

Pregnant women usually should not use aurothioglucose since it has been found to pass through the placenta into the fetus. Women of childbearing age should be aware of the hazards of becoming pregnant while on gold therapy.

Since aurothioglucose can pass into mother's milk, mothers should not breast-feed while taking this drug.

Diabetes and congestive heart failure should be under control before gold therapy begins.

Safety and effectiveness for use of aurothioglucose by children under 6 years old has not been established.

Possible Side Effects

Skin rash and lesions; discoloration of the skin; loss of hair and nails; metallic taste in the mouth; inflammation of the mouth; mouth ulcers; inflammation of the upper respiratory tract; flushing; fainting; dizziness; sweating; vaginitis; rarely, conjunctivitis (inflammation around the eyelid).

Possible Adverse Effects

Fever; cough; shortness of breath; slow heart-beat; swelling of the eyelids or lips; kidney disease;

disorders of the blood; gastritis; colitis; nausea; vomiting; severe stomach pain; stomach cramps; difficulty in swallowing and breathing; loss of appetite. There have been rare reports of disorders affecting the eyes, including inflammation of the iris, corneal ulcers, and gold deposits in eye tissues.

Drug Interactions

Do not use aurothioglucose with penicillamine or antimalarials (i.e., hydroxychloroquine sulfate).

Safety for use of gold compounds with immunosuppressive drugs (i.e., azathioprine and cyclosporine) has not been established.

Usual Dose

Adults: initially 10 mg., followed by second and third doses of 25 mg., then subsequent doses of 50 mg. Initially, doses are administered at intervals of 1 week, followed by intervals of 3 to 4 weeks.

Children (6 to 12 years old): ¼ of adult dosage. Not to exceed 25 mg.

These doses are by injection only and should be administered under a doctor's supervision.

Generic Name
Gold Sodium Thiomalate

Brand Name

Myochrysine

Type of Drug

Gold compound

Prescribed for

Rheumatoid arthritis and juvenile rheumatoid arthritis.

Cautions and Warnings

Do not use gold sodium thiomalate if you have uncontrolled diabetes; kidney or liver disease; a history of infectious hepatitis; marked high blood pressure; heart failure; systemic lupus erythematosus; abnormal blood cells; recently been exposed to radiation; had a severe toxic reaction previously to gold therapy; hives; eczema; colitis; or if you are in a severely debilitated state characterized by very poor circulation to the brain or body.

Notify your doctor if you experience skin rash; loss of hair or nails; inflammation of the mouth; mouth ulcers; metallic taste in the mouth; fever; cough; shortness of breath; fainting; slow heartbeat; thickening of the tongue; difficulty in swallowing and breathing; swelling of the eyelids or lips; nausea; vomiting; stomach cramps; diarrhea; loss of appetite; severe stomach pain. Some of these reactions may be very serious, so it is important that you contact your doctor promptly if you experience any of them.

Skin discoloration and rashes may occur as a result of exposure to sunlight. In addition, careful oral hygiene is important.

Pregnant woman usually should not use gold sodium thiomalate since it has been found to pass through the placenta into the fetus. Women of childbearing age should be aware of the hazards of becoming pregnant while on gold therapy.

Since gold sodium thiomalate can pass into

mother's milk, mothers should not breast-feed while taking this drug.

Diabetes and congestive heart failure should be under control before gold therapy begins.

Possible Side Effects

Skin rash and lesions; discoloration of the skin; loss of hair and nails; metallic taste in the mouth; inflammation of the mouth; mouth ulcers; inflammation of the upper respiratory tract; flushing; fainting; dizziness; sweating; vaginitis; rarely, conjunctivitis.

Possible Adverse Effects

Fever; cough; shortness of breath; slow heartbeat; swelling of the eyelids or lips; kidney disease; disorders of the blood; gastritis; colitis; nausea; vomiting; severe stomach pain; stomach cramps; difficulty in swallowing and breathing; loss of appetite. There have been rare reports of disorders affecting the eyes, including inflammation of the iris, corneal ulcers, and gold deposits in eye tissues.

Drug Interactions

Do not use gold sodium thiomalate with penicillamine or antimalarials (i.e., hydroxychloroquine sulfate).

Safety for use of gold compounds with immunosuppressive drugs (i.e., azathioprine and cyclosporine) has not been established.

Usual Dose

Adults: 10 mg. first injection, then 25 mg., then subsequent injections of 25 mg. to 50 mg. Initially, doses are administered at intervals of 1 week; then, maintenance doses may be spread over intervals ranging from 2 to 20 weeks, or doses may be continued indefinitely.

Children: Initial dose of 10 mg., followed by 1 mg. for every 2.2 lbs. of body weight (not to exceed 50 mg.). The dosage intervals are similar to the adult schedule.

Generic Name
Hydrocortisone

Brand Names

Cortef
Hydrocortone
(Also available in generic form)

Type of Drug

Corticosteroid

Prescribed for

Rheumatoid arthritis; osteoarthritis; ankylosing spondylitis; acute gout; juvenile rheumatoid arthritis; psoriasis; systemic lupus erythematosus; polymyositis; many other nonarthritic conditions.

Cautions and Warnings

Avoid abrupt withdrawal of hydrocortisone. Notify your doctor if, after having your dosage reduced or stopped, you experience fatigue; loss of appetite; weight loss; nausea; vomiting; diarrhea; weakness; dizziness.

Take hydrocortisone with food to avoid upset

stomach. Single daily doses, or every-other-day doses, should be taken preferably before 9:00 A.M. Multiple doses should be spread out evenly throughout the day.

Notify your doctor if you experience unusual weight gain; swelling of the ankles or feet; weakness; black tarry stools; vomiting of blood; heartburn; facial puffiness; menstrual irregularities; prolonged sore throat; fever; cold; infection. (Since hydrocortisone may mask symptoms of infection, it is very important that you report anything that you suspect may be an infection.)

If you are taking hydrocortisone, you should not be vaccinated against infectious diseases.

Pregnant women, women of childbearing potential, and nursing mothers should use hydrocortisone only when the potential benefits clearly outweigh the unknown potential hazards to the fetus. If you become pregnant while taking hydrocortisone, please notify your doctor.

Very stressful situations (such as an accident) may require an increase in dosage.

If you are on long-term hydrocortisone therapy, you should wear or carry identification describing your medication.

If you are sensitive to aspirin or tartrazine, you may be allergic to hydrocortisone.

Use with caution if you suffer from high blood pressure or kidney, liver, thyroid, or heart disease.

Your doctor may prescribe a calcium supplement to help prevent osteoporosis.

Possible Side Effects

Upset stomach; water retention; heart failure; potassium loss; muscle weakness; loss of muscle mass; calcium loss (osteoporosis); slow healing from wounds; black and blue marks; sweating; itching; rash; dizziness; headache.

Possible Adverse Effects

Slowing down of growth in children; depression of the adrenal and/or pituitary glands; diabetes; glaucoma; hypersensitivity or allergic reactions; blood clots; insomnia; weight gain; increased appetite; nausea; feeling of ill health. Psychic derangements may appear, ranging from euphoria to mood swings, personality changes, insomnia, and severe depression.

Drug Interactions

If you are diabetic, hydrocortisone may cause the need for an increase in your antidiabetic medication.

Phenytoin, phenobarbital, rifampin, and possibly ephedrine may cause the need for an alteration in your hydrocortisone dosage.

Hydrocortisone may affect anticoagulant dosages.

Drugs that reduce serum-cholesterol levels, such as cholestyramine and colestipol, may decrease the effects of hydrocortisone.

Interaction with diuretics may cause you to lose potassium. Be aware of signs of lowered potassium levels, such as weakness, muscle cramps, and tiredness, and report them to your doctor. Your doctor may recommend that you eat foods rich in potassium, such as bananas, citrus fruits, melon, and tomatoes.

Use aspirin with caution while taking hydrocortisone.

Usual Dose

Initial dose: 20 to 240 mg. daily. Then adjusted to suit your needs.

Overdosage

Overdosage of hydrocortisone may result in anxiety; depression; confusion; high blood pressure; elevated blood sugar; stomach cramps or bleeding; swelling of the hands or feet; purplish skin patches. If you experience any of these symptoms, contact your doctor immediately, or go to a hospital emergency room. ALWAYS bring the medicine bottle with you.

Generic Name
Hydroxychloroquine Sulfate

Brand Name

Plaquenil Sulfate

Type of Drug

Antimalarial

Prescribed for

Rheumatoid arthritis and discoid and systemic lupus erythematosus.

Cautions and Warnings

Do not use hydroxychloroquine sulfate if you have had an allergic reaction to it or eye problems resulting from similar antimalarial drugs (such as chloroquine hydrochloride).

Hydroxychloroquine sulfate may be fatal if swallowed by a child; keep it out of children's reach at all times.

Use with caution if you suffer from psoriasis, liver disease, or alcoholism.

Notify your doctor if you experience ringing in the ears; hearing loss; fever; sore throat; unusual bleeding or bruising; itching or rash; muscle weakness; bleaching or loss of hair; yellowing of the skin or eyes; emotional changes.

Whenever prolonged therapy is instituted, eye examinations at six month intervals are important, both prior to and during treatment. Any visual disturbance should be reported immediately to your doctor.

Also, periodic blood tests should be performed during prolonged hydroxychloroquine sulfate therapy.

In the treatment of rheumatoid arthritis, hydroxychloroquine sulfate should be discontinued after 6 months if there is no significant improvement in your condition.

The safe use of hydroxychloroquine sulfate in the treatment of juvenile rheumatoid arthritis has not been established.

Pregnant women usually should not use hydroxychloroquine sulfate.

Nursing mothers should use this drug only with their doctor's approval.

To prevent upset stomach, take hydroxychloroquine sulfate with food or milk.

Possible Side Effects

Irritability; headache; nervousness; nightmares; dizziness; uncontrolled eyeball movements; nausea; vomiting; stomach cramps; weakness.

Possible Adverse Effects

Muscle twitches or spasms; convulsions; diarrhea; disorders of blood components; weight loss; serious defects in the eye or field of vision.

Drug Interactions

Using hydroxychloroquine sulfate with phenylbutazone or gold compounds may increase the chance of severe skin reactions.

Avoid using hydroxychloroquine sulfate when taking hepatoxic drugs such as immunosuppressives (i.e., azathioprine).

Usual Dose

Rheumatoid arthritis: Initially 400 to 600 mg. daily. Later, your dosage may be reduced to 200 to 400 mg. daily.

Systemic lupus erythematosus: Initially 400 mg. once or twice daily. Later, your dosage may be reduced to 200 to 400 mg. daily.

Overdosage

Symptoms of hydroxychloroquine sulfate overdose: headache; drowsiness; heart failure; visual disturbances; difficulty in breathing; convulsions. If you think you are experiencing an overdose, contact your doctor immediately, or go to a hospital emergency room. ALWAYS bring the medicine bottle with you.

Generic Name
Ibuprofen

Brand Names

Advil
Motrin
Nuprin
Rufen

Note: Advil and Nuprin are available without prescription in 200 mg. tablets.

Type of Drug

Nonsteroidal anti-inflammatory

Prescribed for

Rheumatoid arthritis, osteoarthritis, relief of mild to moderate pain.

Cautions and Warnings

Do not use ibuprofen if you have had an allergic reaction to aspirin or any other nonsteroidal anti-inflammatory drug (NSAID).

Use with caution if you have a history of kidney, liver, or heart disease; high blood pressure; defects in the blood's clotting ability; or are currently taking anticoagulant medication. If you are suffering from an active peptic ulcer, it is recommended that other forms of drug therapy be tried before using ibuprofen.

With elderly patients, it is recommended that reduced dosages be instituted initially.

Use by pregnant women or nursing mothers is not recommended.

Anemia may occur in patients undergoing long-term therapy with ibuprofen. If you are anemic, it is suggested that you have your hemoglobin values determined frequently.

Pay special attention to any changes in your vision (blurred or partially obstructed vision or color blindness) or any eye complaints that occur when taking ibuprofen. Blurred vision is especially significant and requires a thorough eye examination. It is also recommended that you have your eyes checked regularly if you are undergoing prolonged therapy with ibuprofen.

Avoid aspirin while taking ibuprofen.

Ibuprofen may cause dizziness, drowsiness, or blurred vision; therefore, use caution while driving or performing tasks that require concentration.

To minimize upset stomach, take ibuprofen with food.

Possible Side Effects

Nausea; vomiting; diarrhea; constipation; upset stomach; dizziness; headache; drowsiness; nervousness; insomnia; asthma; heartburn; anemia.

Possible Adverse Effects

Irregular heartbeat; low blood pressure; chest pain; swelling of the hands or feet; adverse effects on the blood; unusual bleeding.

Drug Interactions

Using ibuprofen while taking anticoagulants may require a reduction of anticoagulant medication.

Aspirin may decrease the effectiveness of ibuprofen and probably should not be combined.

Probenecid may enhance the effects of ibuprofen;

therefore, a reduced ibuprofen dosage may be necessary when taking probenecid.

Ibuprofen may increase the effects of anticonvulsants, antidiabetics, and sulfa drugs; your doctor may change the dosages of these other drugs.

Avoid alcohol, since this may increase stomach irritation and drowsiness.

Usual Dose

Rheumatoid arthritis and osteoarthritis: 300 to 600 mg. 3 or 4 times daily.

Mild to moderate pain: 200 mg. every 4 to 6 hours, as necessary.

Safety and effectiveness for children has not been established.

Overdosage

In general, NSAID overdosage is treated by inducing vomiting, followed by the administration of activated charcoal. *However, do NOT induce vomiting or use activated charcoal unless directed to do so by your doctor or poison-control center.* When in doubt, proceed to a hospital emergency room. ALWAYS bring the medicine bottle with you.

Generic Name
Indomethacin

Brand Name

Indocin
(Also available in generic form)

Type of Drug

Nonsteroidal anti-inflammatory

Prescribed for

Rheumatoid arthritis, osteoarthritis, ankylosing spondylitis, acute gout, bursitis, tendinitis.

Cautions and Warnings

Do not use indomethacin if you have had an allergic reaction to aspirin or any other nonsteroidal anti-inflammatory drug (NSAID).

Use with caution if you have a history of kidney, liver, or heart disease; high blood pressure; defects in the blood's clotting ability; or are currently taking anticoagulant medication. If you are suffering from an active peptic ulcer, it is recommended that other forms of drug therapy be tried before using indomethacin.

With elderly patients, it is recommended that reduced dosages be instituted initially.

Use by pregnant women or nursing mothers is not recommended.

Anemia may occur in patients undergoing long-term therapy with indomethacin. If you are anemic, it is suggested that you have your hemoglobin values determined frequently.

Pay special attention to any changes in your vision (blurred or partially obstructed vision or color blindness) or any eye complaints that occur when taking indomethacin. Blurred vision is especially significant and requires a thorough eye examination. It is also recommended that you have your eyes checked regularly if you are undergoing prolonged therapy with indomethacin.

Avoid aspirin while taking indomethacin.

Indomethacin may cause dizziness, drowsiness, or blurred vision; therefore, use caution while driving or performing tasks that require concentration.

Indomethacin should be used with extreme caution in the presence of infection, since this drug may mask the usual signs of infection.

To minimize upset stomach, take indomethacin with food.

Possible Side Effects

Nausea; vomiting; diarrhea; constipation; upset stomach; dizziness; headache; drowsiness; nervousness; insomnia; asthma; heartburn; anemia.

In addition, indomethacin may aggravate preexisting psychiatric disturbances, epilepsy, Parkinson's disease, or kidney impairment.

Possible Adverse Effects

Irregular heartbeat; low blood pressure; chest pain; swelling of the hands or feet; adverse effects on the blood; unusual bleeding.

Drug Interactions

Using indomethacin while taking anticoagulants may require a reduction of anticoagulant medication.

Aspirin may decrease the effectiveness of indomethacin and probably should not be combined.

Probenecid may enhance the effects of indomethacin; therefore, a reduced indomethacin dosage may be necessary when taking probenecid.

Indomethacin may increase the effects of anticonvulsants, antidiabetics, and sulfa drugs; your doctor may change the dosages of these other drugs.

Avoid alcohol, since this may increase stomach irritation and drowsiness.

Indomethacin may also block the effects of anti-hypertensive medications like diuretics and beta blockers.

Use lithium with caution when taking indomethacin.

Using triamterene with indomethacin may result in kidney failure.

Usual Dose

Rheumatoid arthritis, osteoarthritis, ankylosing spondylitis: 25 mg. 2 or 3 times daily (or 75 mg. of Indocin SR—a sustained-release capsule—once daily). Dosage may be increased to 200 mg. daily.

Acute gout: 50 mg. 3 times daily until pain subsides. Then rapidly reduce dosage. (The sustained-release capsule—Indocin SR—should not be used to treat acute gout.)

Bursitis tendinitis: 75 to 100 mg. daily.

Indomethacin should not be used as a simple pain reliever for mild to moderate pain.

Not recommended for children under the age of 14.

Overdosage

In general, NSAID overdosage is treated by inducing vomiting, followed by the administration of activated charcoal. *However, do NOT induce vomiting or use activated charcoal unless directed to do so by your doctor or poison-control center.* When in doubt, proceed to a hospital emergency room. ALWAYS bring the medicine bottle with you.

Generic Name
Meclofenamate Sodium

Brand Name

Meclomen

Type of Drug

Nonsteroidal anti-inflammatory

Prescribed for

Rheumatoid arthritis, osteoarthritis.

Cautions and Warnings

Do not use meclofenamate sodium if you have had an allergic reaction to aspirin or any other nonsteroidal anti-inflammatory drug (NSAID).

Use with caution if you have a history of kidney, liver, or heart disease; high blood pressure; defects in the blood's clotting ability; or are currently taking anticoagulant medication. If you are suffering from an active peptic ulcer, it is recommended that other forms of drug therapy be tried before using meclofenamate sodium.

With elderly patients, it is recommended that reduced dosages be instituted initially.

Use by pregnant women or nursing mothers is not recommended.

Anemia may occur in patients undergoing long-term therapy with meclofenamate sodium. If you are anemic, it is suggested that you have your hemoglobin values determined frequently.

Pay special attention to any changes in your vision (blurred or partially obstructed vision or color blindness) or any eye complaints that occur when taking meclofenamate sodium. Blurred vision is especially significant and requires a thorough eye examination. It is also recommended that you have your eyes checked regularly if you are undergoing prolonged therapy with meclofenamate sodium.

Avoid aspirin while taking meclofenamate sodium.

Meclofenamate sodium may cause dizziness, drowsiness, or blurred vision; therefore, use caution while driving or performing tasks that require concentration.

To minimize upset stomach, take meclofenamate sodium with food.

Possible Side Effects

Nausea; vomiting; diarrhea; constipation; upset stomach; dizziness; headache; drowsiness; nervousness; insomnia; asthma; heartburn; anemia.

Possible Adverse Effects

Irregular heartbeat; low blood pressure; chest pain; swelling of the hands or feet; adverse effects on the blood; unusual bleeding.

Drug Interactions

Using meclofenamate sodium while taking anticoagulants may require a reduction of anticoagulant medication.

Aspirin may decrease the effectiveness of meclofenamate sodium and probably should not be combined.

Probenecid may enhance the effects of meclofenamate sodium; therefore, a reduced meclofenamate sodium dosage may be necessary when taking probenecid.

Meclofenamate sodium may increase the effects of anticonvulsants, antidiabetics, and sulfa drugs; your doctor may change the dosages of these other drugs.

Avoid alcohol, since this may increase stomach irritation and drowsiness.

Meclofenamate sodium enhances the effects of warfarin; therefore, the dosage of warfarin should be reduced when given with meclofenamate sodium.

Usual Dose

200 to 400 mg. daily in 3 or 4 equal doses. 2 to 3 weeks may be necessary before benefits of drug therapy are evident.

Not recommended for use by children.

Overdosage

In general, NSAID overdosage is treated by inducing vomiting, followed by the administration of activated charcoal. *However, do NOT induce vomiting or use activated charcoal unless directed to do so by your doctor or poison-control center.* When in doubt, proceed to a hospital emergency room. ALWAYS bring the medicine bottle with you.

Generic Name
Mefenamic Acid

Brand Name

Ponstel

Type of Drug

Nonsteroidal anti-inflammatory

Prescribed for

Relief of mild to moderate pain.

Cautions and Warnings

Do not use mefenamic acid if you have had an allergic reaction to aspirin or any other nonsteroidal anti-inflammatory drug (NSAID).

Use with caution if you have a history of kidney, liver, or heart disease; high blood pressure; defects in the blood's clotting ability; or are currently taking anticoagulant medication. If you are suffering from an active peptic ulcer, it is recommended that other forms of drug therapy be tried before using mefenamic acid.

With elderly patients, it is recommended that reduced dosages be instituted initially.

Use by pregnant women or nursing mothers is not recommended.

Anemia may occur in patients undergoing long-term therapy with mefenamic acid. If you are anemic, it is suggested that you have your hemoglobin values determined frequently.

Pay special attention to any changes in your vision (blurred or partially obstructed vision or color blindness) or any eye complaints that occur when taking mefenamic acid. Blurred vision is especially significant and requires a thorough eye examination. It is also recommended that you have your eyes checked regularly if you are undergoing prolonged therapy with mefenamic acid.

Avoid aspirin while taking mefenamic acid.

Mefenamic acid may cause dizziness, drowsiness, or blurred vision; therefore, use caution while driving or performing tasks that require concentration.

Do not use mefenamic acid if you have a history of seriously impaired kidney function.

Do not use mefenamic acid if you suffer from ulcers or other chronic inflammations of the stomach.

To minimize upset stomach, take mefenamic acid with food.

Possible Side Effects

Nausea; vomiting; diarrhea; constipation; upset stomach; dizziness; headache; drowsiness; nervousness; insomnia; asthma; heartburn; anemia.

Possible Adverse Effects

Irregular heartbeat; low blood pressure; chest pain; swelling of the hands or feet; adverse effects on the blood; unusual bleeding.

Drug Interactions

Using mefenamic acid while taking anticoagulants may require a reduction of anticoagulant medication.

Aspirin may decrease the effectiveness of mefenamic acid and probably should not be combined.

Probenecid may enhance the effects of mefenamic acid; therefore, a reduced mefenamic acid dosage may be necessary when taking probenecid.

Mefenamic acid may increase the effects of anticonvulsants, antidiabetics, and sulfa drugs; your doctor may change the dosages of these other drugs.

Avoid alcohol, since this may increase stomach irritation and drowsiness.

Usual Dose

Adults and children over 14: Initially 500 mg., then 250 mg. every 6 hours as needed.

Overdosage

In general, NSAID overdosage is treated by inducing vomiting, followed by the administration of activated charcoal. *However, do NOT induce vomiting or use activated charcoal unless directed to do so by your doctor or poison-control center.* When in doubt, proceed to a hospital emergency room. ALWAYS bring the medicine bottle with you.

Generic Name
Methylprednisolone

Brand Name

Medrol
(Also available in generic form)

Type of Drug

Corticosteroid

Prescribed for

Rheumatoid arthritis; osteoarthritis; ankylosing spondylitis; acute gout; juvenile rheumatoid arthritis; psoriasis; systemic lupus erythematosus; polymyositis; many other nonarthritic conditions.

Cautions and Warnings

Avoid abrupt withdrawal of methylprednisolone. Notify your doctor if, after having your dosage reduced or stopped, you experience fatigue; loss of appetite; weight loss; nausea; vomiting; diarrhea; weakness; dizziness.

Take methylprednisolone with food to avoid upset stomach. Single daily doses, or every-other-day doses, should be taken preferably before 9:00 A.M. Multiple doses should be spread out evenly throughout the day.

Notify your doctor if you experience unusual weight gain; swelling of the ankles or feet; weakness; black tarry stools; vomiting of blood; heartburn; facial puffiness; menstrual irregularities; prolonged sore throat; fever; cold; infection. (Since methylprednisolone may mask symptoms of infection, it is very important that you report anything that you suspect may be an infection.)

If you are taking methylprednisolone, you should not be vaccinated against infectious diseases.

Pregnant women, women of childbearing potential, and nursing mothers should use methylprednisolone only when the potential benefits clearly outweigh the unknown potential hazards to the fetus. If you become pregnant while taking methylprednisolone, please notify your doctor.

Very stressful situations (such as an accident) may require an increase in dosage.

If you are on long-term methylprednisolone therapy, you should wear or carry identification describing your medication.

If you are sensitive to aspirin or tartrazine, you may be allergic to methylprednisolone.

Use with caution if you suffer from high blood pressure or kidney, liver, thyroid, or heart disease.

Your doctor may prescribe a calcium supplement to help prevent osteoporosis.

Possible Side Effects

Upset stomach; water retention; heart failure; potassium loss; muscle weakness; loss of muscle mass; calcium loss (osteoporosis); slow healing from wounds; black and blue marks; sweating; itching; rash; dizziness; headache.

Possible Adverse Effects

Slowing down of growth in children; depression of the adrenal and/or pituitary glands; diabetes; glaucoma; hypersensitivity or allergic reactions; blood clots; insomnia; weight gain; increased appetite; nausea; feeling of ill health. Psychic derangements may appear, ranging from euphoria to mood swings, personality changes, insomnia, and severe depression.

Drug Interactions

If you are diabetic, methylprednisolone may cause the need for an increase in your antidiabetic medication.

Phenytoin, phenobarbital, rifampin, and possibly ephedrine may cause the need for an alteration in your methylprednisolone dosage.

Methylprednisolone may affect anticoagulant dosages.

Drugs that reduce serum-cholesterol levels, such as cholestyramine and colestipol, may decrease the effects of methylprednisolone.

Interaction with diuretics may cause you to lose potassium. Be aware of signs of lowered potassium levels, such as weakness, muscle cramps, and tiredness, and report them to your doctor. Your doctor may recommend that you eat foods rich in potassium, such as bananas, citrus fruits, melon, and tomatoes.

Use aspirin with caution while taking methyl-prednisolone.

Usual Dose

Initial dose: 4 to 48 mg. daily. Then adjusted to suit your needs.

Overdosage

Overdosage of methylprednisolone may result in anxiety; depression; confusion; high blood pressure; elevated blood sugar; stomach cramps or bleeding; swelling of the hands or feet; purplish skin patches. If you experience any of these symptoms, contact your doctor immediately, or go to a hospital emergency room. ALWAYS bring the medicine bottle with you.

Generic Names
Naproxen
Naproxen Sodium

Brand Names

Anaprox (naproxen sodium)
Naprosyn (naproxen)

Type of Drug

Nonsteroidal anti-inflammatory

Prescribed for

Rheumatoid arthritis, osteoarthritis, ankylosing

spondylitis, acute gout, relief of mild to moderate pain.

Cautions and Warnings

Do not use naproxen (or naproxen sodium) if you have had an allergic reaction to aspirin or any other nonsteroidal anti-inflammatory drug (NSAID).

Use with caution if you have a history of kidney, liver, or heart disease; high blood pressure; defects in the blood's clotting ability; or are currently taking anticoagulant medication. If you are suffering from an active peptic ulcer, it is recommended that other forms of drug therapy be tried before using naproxen (or naproxen sodium).

With elderly patients, it is recommended that reduced dosages be instituted initially.

Use by pregnant women or nursing mothers is not recommended.

Anemia may occur in patients undergoing long-term therapy with naproxen (or naproxen sodium). If you are anemic, it is suggested that you have your hemoglobin values determined frequently.

Pay special attention to any changes in your vision (blurred or partially obstructed vision or color blindness) or any eye complaints that occur when taking naproxen (or naproxen sodium). Blurred vision is especially significant and requires a thorough eye examination. It is also recommended that you have your eyes checked regularly if you are undergoing prolonged therapy with naproxen (or naproxen sodium).

Avoid aspirin while taking naproxen (or naproxen sodium).

Naproxen (or naproxen sodium) may cause dizziness, drowsiness, or blurred vision; therefore, use caution while driving or performing tasks that require concentration.

To minimize upset stomach, take naproxen (or naproxen sodium) with food.

Possible Side Effects

Nausea; vomiting; diarrhea; constipation; upset stomach; dizziness; headache; drowsiness; nervousness; insomnia; asthma; heartburn; anemia.

Possible Adverse Effects

Irregular heartbeat; low blood pressure; chest pain; swelling of the hands or feet; adverse effects on the blood; unusual bleeding.

Drug Interactions

Using naproxen (or naproxen sodium) while taking anticoagulants may require a reduction of anticoagulant medication.

Aspirin may decrease the effectiveness of naproxen (or naproxen sodium) and should probably not be combined.

Probenecid may enhance the effects of naproxen (or naproxen sodium); therefore, a reduced naproxen (or naproxen sodium) dosage may be necessary when taking probenecid.

Naproxen (or naproxen sodium) may increase the effects of anticonvulsants, antidiabetics, and sulfa drugs; your doctor may change the dosages of these other drugs.

Avoid alcohol, since this may increase stomach irritation and drowsiness.

Usual Dose

Rheumatoid arthritis, osteoarthritis, ankylosing spondylitis: 250 to 375 mg. Naprosyn (or 275 mg. Anaprox) twice daily.

Acute gout: 750 mg. Naprosyn (or 825 mg. Anaprox), followed by 250 mg. Naprosyn (or 275 mg. Anaprox) every 8 hours until pain subsides.

Mild to moderate pain: 500 mg. Naprosyn (or 550 mg. Anaprox), followed by 250 mg. Naprosyn (or 275 mg. Anaprox) every 6 to 8 hours.

Safety and effectiveness for use by children has not been established.

Overdosage

In general, NSAID overdosage is treated by inducing vomiting, followed by the administration of activated charcoal. *However, do NOT induce vomiting or use activated charcoal unless directed to do so by your doctor or poison-control center.* When in doubt, proceed to a hospital emergency room. ALWAYS bring the medicine bottle with you.

Generic Name

Oxycodone Hydrochloride with Acetaminophen

Brand Names

Percocet
Tylox

Type of Drug

Narcotic pain reliever combined with nonprescription pain reliever

Prescribed for

Relief of mild to moderate pain.

Cautions and Warnings

Do not take this drug if you know you are allergic or sensitive to any of its components. Use oxycodone hydrochloride with acetaminophen with extreme caution if you suffer from asthma or other breathing problems. Long-term use of this drug may cause drug dependence or addiction. The oxycodone hydrochloride ingredient is a respiratory depressant and affects the central nervous system, producing sleepiness, tiredness, and/or inability to concentrate. Be careful if you are driving, operating machinery, or performing other functions that require concentration. If you are pregnant or suspect that you are pregnant, do not take this drug.

Oxycodone hydrochloride with acetaminophen is best taken with food to prevent stomach upset.

Possible Side Effects

Most frequent: light-headedness; dizziness; sleepiness; nausea; vomiting; loss of appetite; sweating. If these occur, ask your doctor about lowering your dose of oxycodone hydrochloride with acetaminophen. Usually the side effects disappear if you simply lie down.

If you experience shallow breathing or difficulty in breathing, call your doctor or got to the hospital.

Possible Adverse Effects

Adverse effects include euphoria (feeling high); weakness; sleepiness; headache; agitation; uncoordinated muscle movement; minor hallucinations; disorientation and visual disturbances; dry mouth; loss of appetite; constipation; flushing of the face; rapid heartbeat; palpitations; faintness; urinary difficulties or hesitancy; reduced sex drive and/or potency; itching; rash; anemia; lowered blood sugar; yellowing of the skin and/or whites of the eyes. Narcotic pain relievers may aggravate convulsions in those who have had convulsions in the past.

Drug Interactions

Because of its depressant effect and potential effect on breathing, oxycodone hydrochloride with acetaminophen should be taken with extreme care in combination with alcohol, sleeping medicine, tranquilizers, or other depressant drugs.

Dependence and Addiction

Most people are aware that narcotics have an extremely high potential for abuse and addiction. This varies according to the strength of the particular drug, frequency of use, the circumstances under which it is used, and the individual's susceptibility to addiction.

It is very important that you inform your doctor about any problems that you or any member of your family has had with alcohol or tranquilizers.

Dependence to narcotics manifests itself through increased tolerance to drug's pain relief; if you notice that the pain won't go away unless you increase your dosage, you may be becoming dependent on the narcotic.

The major signs of addiction include varying degrees of anxiety when the drug is suddenly withdrawn.

Withdrawal Symptoms

Yawning; excessive sweating; sneezing; twitching and kicking; tremors; gooseflesh; fever and chills alternating with flushing; anxiety; dilated pupils; over-all weakness and aches; loss of appetite; nausea; vomiting; diarrhea; cramps.

Withdrawal Treatment

Treatment for narcotic withdrawal, which should be handled *only* by trained medical personnel, often includes the use of sedatives to ease anxiety, after which the narcotic is gradually withdrawn over a period of several days.

Usual Dose

Adults: 1 tablet every 6 hours.
Children: Not recommended for children.

Overdosage

Symptoms are depression of respiration (breathing); extreme tiredness progressing to stupor and then coma; pinpointed pupils of the eyes; no response to stimulation such as a pinprick; cold and clammy skin; slowing of the heart rate; lowering of blood pressure; yellowing of the skin and/or whites of the eyes; bluish color in skin of hands and feet; fever; excitement; delirium; convulsions; cardiac arrest; liver toxicity (shown by nausea, vomiting, pain in the abdomen, and diarrhea). If you think you are experiencing an overdose, go to a hospital emergency room immediately. ALWAYS bring the medicine bottle with you.

Generic Name

Oxycodone Hydrochloride with Aspirin

Brand Names

Codoxy
Percodan

Type of Drug

Narcotic pain reliever combined with nonprescription pain reliever

Prescribed for

Relief of mild to moderate pain.

Cautions and Warnings

Do not take this drug if you know you are allergic or sensitive to any of its components. Use oxycodone hydrochloride with aspirin with extreme caution if you suffer from asthma or other breathing problems. Long-term use of this drug may cause drug dependence or addiction. The oxycodone hydrochloride ingredient is a respiratory depressant and affects the central nervous system, producing sleepiness, tiredness, and/or inability to concentrate. If you are pregnant or suspect that you are pregnant, do not take this drug.

Drowsiness may occur: be careful when driving or operating hazardous machinery.

Oxycodone hydrochloride with aspirin is best taken with food to prevent stomach upset.

Possible Side Effects

Most frequent: light-headedness; dizziness;

sleepiness; nausea; vomiting; loss of appetite; sweating. If these occur, ask your doctor about lowering your dosage of oxycodone hydrochloride with aspirin. Usually the side effects disappear if you simply lie down.

If you experience shallow breathing or difficulty in breathing, call your doctor or go to the hospital.

Possible Adverse Effects

Euphoria (feeling high); weakness; sleepiness; headache; agitation; uncoordinated muscle movement; minor hallucinations; disorientation and visual disturbances; dry mouth; loss of appetite; constipation; flushing of the face; rapid heartbeat; palpitations; faintness; urinary difficulties or hesitancy; reduced sex drive and/or potency; itching; skin rash; anemia; lowered blood sugar; yellowing of the skin and/or whites of the eyes. Narcotic pain relievers may aggravate convulsions in those who have had convulsions in the past.

Drug Interactions

Interaction with alcohol, tranquilizers, barbiturates, or sleeping pills produces tiredness, sleepiness, or inability to concentrate, and seriously increases the depressive effect of this drug.

The aspirin ingredient can affect anticoagulant (blood-thinning) therapy. Be sure to discuss this with your doctor so that the proper dosage adjustment can be made.

Interaction with corticosteroids, phenylbutazone, or alcohol can cause severe stomach irritation with possible bleeding.

Dependence and Addiction

Most people are aware that narcotics have an extremely high potential for abuse and addiction. This varies according to the strength of the particular drug, frequency of use, the circumstances under which it is used, and the individual's susceptibility to addiction.

It is very important that you inform your doctor about any problems that you or any member of your family has had with alcohol or tranquilizers.

Dependence to narcotics manifests itself through increased tolerance to the drug's pain relief; if you notice that the pain won't go away unless you increase your dosage, you may be becoming dependent on the narcotic.

The major signs of addiction include varying degrees of anxiety when the drug is suddenly withdrawn.

Withdrawal Symptoms

Yawning; excessive sweating; sneezing; twitching and kicking; tremors; gooseflesh; fever and chills alternating with flushing; anxiety; dilated pupils; over-all weakness and aches; loss of appetite; nausea; vomiting; diarrhea; cramps.

Withdrawal Treatment

Treatment for narcotic withdrawal, which should be handled *only* by trained medical personnel, often includes the use of sedatives to ease anxiety, after which the narcotic is gradually withdrawn over a period of several days.

Usual Dose

Adults: 1 tablet every 6 hours as needed for relief of pain.
Children: Not recommended for children.

Overdosage

Symptoms are depression of respiration (breathing); extreme tiredness progressing to stupor and then coma; pinpointed pupils of the eyes; no response to stimulation such as a pinprick; cold and clammy skin; slowing down of the heartbeat; lowering of blood pressure; convulsions; cardiac arrest. If you think you are experiencing an overdose, go to a hospital emergency room immediately. ALWAYS bring the medicine bottle with you.

Generic Names
Oxyphenbutazone
Phenylbutazone

Brand Names

Oxalid (oxyphenbutazone)
Tandearil (oxyphenbutazone)
Azolid (phenylbutazone)
Butazolidin (phenylbutazone)
(Phenylbutazone is also available in generic form)

Type of Drug

Nonsteroidal anti-inflammatory

Prescribed for

Acute gouty arthritis; rheumatoid arthritis; osteoarthritis; ankylosing spondylitis.

Cautions and Warnings

Do not take these drugs if you have a history of

or symptoms associated with gastrointestinal inflammation of ulcer, including severe, recurrent, or persistent upset stomach; asthma; thyroid disease; high blood pressure; inflammation of the mouth; severe kidney, heart, or liver disease; temporal arteritis; pancreatitis.

Also, use by pregnant women, children (14 years or younger), nursing mothers, or senile patients should be avoided.

Oxyphenbutazone and phenylbutazone should not be prescribed until a careful and detailed history, plus physical and laboratory tests, have been completed by a doctor. If your problem can be treated by a less-toxic drug, such as aspirin, use that first. *Never* take more than the recommended dosage: this could lead to toxic effects. If the drug is not effective after 1 week, inform your doctor.

If you have fever, sore throat, mouth sores, unusual bleeding or bruising, blurred vision, black or tarry stools, unusual weight gain, swelling of the legs or feet, or skin rash, report this to your doctor immediately.

Oxyphenbutazone and phenylbutazone can cause drowsiness: be careful when driving or performing tasks that require concentration. Never take alcohol while taking these drugs.

To prevent upset stomach, take these drugs with food. If stomach pain persists, contact your doctor.

Possible Side Effects

Most common: stomach upset; drowsiness; water retention; heartburn; indigestion.

Possible Adverse Effects

Infrequent: acute gastric or duodenal ulcer; ulceration or perforation of the large bowel; bleeding from the stomach; anemia; stomach pain; vomiting; nausea; diarrhea; changes in the components of the blood; disruption of the normal chemical balance of the body. These drugs can cause fatal or nonfatal hepatitis; black and blue marks on the skin; drug allergy; itching; serious rashes; fever; signs of arthritis. They have been known to cause kidney effects including bleeding and kidney stones. Also, they can cause heart disease; high blood pressure; blurred vision; bleeding in the eye; detached retina; hearing loss; high blood sugar; thyroid disease; agitation; confusion; lethargy.

Drug Interactions

Oxyphenbutazone and phenylbutazone increase the effects of blood-thinning drugs, phenytoin, insulin, and oral antidiabetic agents. If you are taking any of these drugs, alert your doctor immediately.

Using phenylbutazone with digitoxin may decrease the effects of digitoxin. On the other hand, discontinuing phenylbutazone may lead to digitoxin toxicity.

Usual Dose

Adults: For rheumatoid arthritis, ankylosing spondylitis, osteoarthritis, initial daily dose is 300 to 600 mg. divided into 3 or 4 equal doses for 7 days. Maintenance dose may range from 100 to 400 mg. daily.

For acute gouty arthritis: Initial dose of 400 mg. followed by 100 mg. every 4 hours. Therapy should not exceed 7 days.

Elderly (60 years and over): Drug to be given

only for 7 days because of high risk of severe reactions. Not to be given to senile patients.

Overdosage

Symptoms include convulsions; euphoria; depression; headache; hallucinations; giddiness; ringing in the ears; difficulty in hearing; dizziness; water retention; coma; rapid breathing; insomnia. If you think you are experiencing an overdose, contact your doctor immediately, or go to a hospital emergency room. ALWAYS bring the medicine bottle with you.

Generic Name
Paramethasone Acetate

Brand Name

Haldrone

Type of Drug

Corticosteroid

Prescribed for

Rheumatoid arthritis; osteoarthritis; ankylosing spondylitis; acute gout; juvenile rheumatoid arthritis; psoriasis; systemic lupus erythematosus; polymyositis; many other nonarthritic conditions.

Cautions and Warnings

Avoid abrupt withdrawal of paramethasone acetate. Notify your doctor if, after having your dosage reduced or stopped, you experience fatigue;

loss of appetite; weight loss; nausea; vomiting; diarrhea; weakness; dizziness.

Take paramethasone acetate with food to avoid upset stomach. Single daily doses, or every-other-day doses, should be taken preferably before 9:00 A.M. Multiple doses should be spread out evenly throughout the day.

Notify your doctor if you experience unusual weight gain; swelling of the ankles or feet; weakness; black tarry stools; vomiting of blood; heartburn; facial puffiness; menstrual irregularities; prolonged sore throat; fever; cold; infection. (Since paramethasone acetate may mask symptoms of infection, it is very important that you report anything that you suspect may be an infection.)

If you are taking paramethasone acetate, you should not be vaccinated against infectious diseases.

Pregnant women, women of childbearing potential, and nursing mothers should use paramethasone acetate only when the potential benefits clearly outweigh the unknown potential hazards to the fetus. If you become pregnant while taking paramethasone acetate, please notify your doctor.

Very stressful situations (such as an accident) may require an increase in dosage.

If you are on long-term paramethasone acetate therapy, you should wear or carry identification describing your medication.

If you are sensitive to aspirin or tartrazine, you may be allergic to paramethasone acetate.

Use with caution if you suffer from high blood pressure or kidney, liver, thyroid, or heart disease.

Your doctor may prescribe a calcium supplement to help prevent osteoporosis.

Possible Side Effects

Upset stomach; water retention; heart failure; potassium loss; muscle weakness; loss of muscle mass; calcium loss (osteoporosis); slow healing from wounds; black and blue marks; sweating; itching; rash; dizziness; headache.

Possible Adverse Effects

Slowing down of growth in children; depression of the adrenal and/or pituitary glands; diabetes; glaucoma; hypersensitivity or allergic reactions; blood clots; insomnia; weight gain; increased appetite; nausea; feeling of ill health. Psychic derangements may appear, ranging from euphoria to mood swings, personality changes, insomnia, and severe depression.

Drug Interactions

If you are diabetic, paramethasone acetate may cause the need for an increase in your antidiabetic medication.

Phenytoin, phenobarbital, rifampin, and possibly ephedrine may cause the need for an alteration in your paramethasone acetate dosage.

Paramethasone acetate may affect anticoagulant dosages.

Drugs that reduce serum-cholesterol levels, such as cholestyramine and colestipol, may decrease the effects of paramethasone acetate.

Interaction with diuretics may cause you to lose potassium. Be aware of signs of lowered potassium levels, such as weakness, muscle cramps, and tiredness, and report them to your doctor. Your doctor may recommend that you take a potassium supplement, or that you eat foods rich in potassium, such as bananas, citrus fruits, melon, and tomatoes.

Use aspirin with caution while taking parameth-asone acetate.

Usual Dose

Initial dose: 2 to 24 mg. daily. Then adjusted to suit your needs.

Overdosage

Overdosage of paramethasone acetate may result in anxiety; depression; confusion; high blood pressure; elevated blood sugar; stomach cramps or bleeding; swelling of the hands or feet; purplish skin patches. If you experience any of these symptoms, contact your doctor immediately, or go to a hospital emergency room. ALWAYS bring the medicine bottle with you.

Generic Name
Penicillamine

Brand Names

Cuprimine
Depen Titratabs

Type of Drug

Penicillamine

Prescribed for

Severe, active rheumatoid arthritis that has not responded to other treatment.

Cautions and Warnings

Do not take penicillamine if you have a history of or suffer from kidney disease.

Do not take penicillamine if you are pregnant. Women of childbearing age should be warned of the potential dangers to the developing fetus. You should report promptly to your doctor any missed menstrual periods or any signs of possible pregnancy.

Safety for use by breast-feeding mothers has not been established.

Routine urinalysis, blood tests, and platelet counts should be done every two weeks for the first six months of therapy and monthly thereafter. Periodic liver-function tests should be done.

Notify your doctor if you experience skin rash; unusual bleeding or bruising; sore throat; shortness of breath; unexplained coughing or wheezing; fever; chills; sense of ill health.

Two or three months may pass before you notice any benefits from taking penicillamine.

Take penicillamine on an empty stomach, one hour before, or two hours after, meals (and at least one hour apart from any other drug, food, or milk).

Possible Side Effects

Drug fever (usually in the second or third week of therapy); rash (usually during the first few months of treatment); loss of appetite; loss of taste sensation; heartburn.

Possible Adverse Effects

Lupuslike symptoms; nausea; vomiting; diarrhea; mouth sores; colitis; kidney, liver, or blood disorders.

Drug Interactions

Do not use penicillamine if you are taking anti-malarial or cytotoxic drugs, oxyphenbutazone, phenylbutazone, or gold therapy.

The effects of penicillamine are markedly decreased by food, antacids, or iron salts. Avoid taking these simultaneously with penicillamine.

Penicillamine may decrease the effects of digoxin, which may result in the need to adjust your digoxin dosage.

Usual Dose

Initial dose: 125 to 250 mg. once daily. Increased by 125 or 250 mg. daily at 1- to 3-month intervals until benefits appear.

Maintenance dose: Adjusted to suit your needs. However, some patients respond to 500 to 750 mg. daily, or less. After 2 years, most patients will require a 1000 mg. dose.

Generic Name
Piroxicam

Brand Name

Feldene

Type of Drug

Nonsteroidal anti-inflammatory

Prescribed for

Rheumatoid arthritis, osteoarthritis.

Cautions and Warnings

Do not use piroxicam if you have had an allergic reaction to aspirin or any other nonsteroidal anti-inflammatory drug (NSAID).

Use with caution if you have a history of kidney, liver, or heart disease; high blood pressure; defects in the blood's clotting ability; or are currently taking anticoagulant medication. If you are suffering from an active peptic ulcer, it is recommended that other forms of drug therapy be tried before using piroxicam.

With elderly patients, it is recommended that reduced dosages be instituted initially.

Use by pregnant women or nursing mothers is not recommended.

Anemia may occur in patients undergoing long-term therapy with piroxicam. If you are anemic, it is suggested that you have your hemoglobin values determined frequently.

Pay special attention to any changes in your vision (blurred or partially obstructed vision or color blindness) or any eye complaints that occur when taking piroxicam. Blurred vision is especially significant and requires a thorough eye examination. It is also recommended that you have your eyes checked regularly if you are undergoing prolonged therapy with piroxicam.

Avoid aspirin while taking piroxicam.

Piroxicam may cause dizziness, drowsiness, or blurred vision; therefore, use caution while driving or performing tasks that require concentration.

To minimize upset stomach, take piroxicam with food.

Possible Side Effects

Nausea; vomiting; diarrhea; constipation; upset stomach; dizziness; headache; drowsiness;
nervousness; insomnia; asthma; heartburn; anemia.

Possible Adverse Effects

Irregular heartbeat; low blood pressure; chest
pain; swelling of the hands or feet; adverse effects on the blood; unusual bleeding.

Drug Interactions

Using piroxicam while taking anticoagulants may
require a reduction of anticoagulant medication.
Aspirin may decrease the effectiveness of piroxicam and probably should not be combined.
Probenecid may enhance the effects of piroxicam;
therefore, a reduced piroxicam dosage may be
necessary when taking probenecid.
Piroxicam may increase the effects of anticonvulsants, antidiabetics, and sulfa drugs; your doctor may change the dosages of these other drugs.
Avoid alcohol, since this may increase stomach
irritation and drowsiness.

Usual Dose

Adult: 20 mg. daily (maximum dose).
Children: Safety and effectiveness for use by
children has not been established.

Overdosage

In general, NSAID overdosage is treated by inducing vomiting, followed by the administration of
activated charcoal. *However, do NOT induce vomit-*

ing or use activated charcoal unless directed to do so by your doctor or poison-control center. When in doubt, proceed to a hospital emergency room. ALWAYS bring the medicine bottle with you.

Generic Name

Prednisolone

Brand Names

Cortalone
Delta-Cortef
Fernisolone-P
Predoxine-5
Sterane
(Also available in generic form)

Type of Drug

Corticosteroid

Prescribed for

Rheumatoid arthritis; osteoarthritis; ankylosing spondylitis; acute gout; juvenile rheumatoid arthritis; psoriasis; systemic lupus erythematosus; polymyositis; many other nonarthritic conditions.

Cautions and Warnings

Avoid abrupt withdrawal of prednisolone. Notify your doctor if, after having your dosage reduced or stopped, you experience fatigue; loss of appetite; weight loss; nausea; vomiting; diarrhea; weakness; dizziness.

Take prednisolone with food to avoid upset stomach. Single daily doses, or every-other-day doses, should be taken preferably before 9:00 A.M. Multiple doses should be spread out evenly throughout the day.

Notify your doctor if you experience unusual weight gain; swelling of the ankles or feet; weakness; black tarry stools; vomiting of blood; heartburn; facial puffiness; menstrual irregularities; prolonged sore throat; fever; cold; infection. (Since prednisolone may mask symptoms of infection, it is very important that you report anything that you suspect may be an infection.)

If you are taking prednisolone, you should not be vaccinated against infectious diseases.

Pregnant women, women of childbearing potential, and nursing mothers should use prednisolone only when the potential benefits clearly outweigh the unknown potential hazards to the fetus. If you become pregnant while taking prednisolone, please notify your doctor.

Very stressful situations (such as an accident) may require an increase in dosage.

If you are on long-term prednisolone therapy, you should wear or carry identification describing your medication.

If you are sensitive to aspirin or tartrazine, you may be allergic to prednisolone.

Use with caution if you suffer from high blood pressure or kidney, liver, thyroid, or heart disease.

Your doctor may prescribe a calcium supplement to help prevent osteoporosis.

Possible Side Effects

Upset stomach; water retention; heart failure; potassium loss; muscle weakness; loss of muscle mass; calcium loss (osteoporosis); slow healing from wounds; black and blue marks; sweating; itching; rash; dizziness; headache.

Possible Adverse Effects

Slowing down of growth in children; depression of the adrenal and/or pituitary glands; diabetes; glaucoma; hypersensitivity or allergic reactions; blood clots; insomnia; weight gain; increased appetite; nausea; feeling of ill health. Psychic derangements may appear, ranging from euphoria to mood swings, personality changes, insomnia, and severe depression.

Drug Interactions

If you are diabetic, prednisolone may cause the need for an increase in your antidiabetic medication.

Phenytoin, phenobarbital, rifampin, and possibly ephedrine may cause the need for an alteration in your prednisolone dosage.

Prednisolone may affect anticoagulant dosages.

Drugs that reduce serum-cholesterol levels, such as cholestyramine and colestipol, may decrease the effects of prednisolone.

Interaction with diuretics may cause you to lose potassium. Be aware of signs of lowered potassium levels, such as weakness, muscle cramps, and tiredness, and report them to your doctor. Your doctor may recommend that you take a potassium supplement, or that you eat foods rich in potassium, such as bananas, citrus fruits, melon, and tomatoes.

Use aspirin with caution while taking prednisolone.

Usual Dose

Initial dose: 5 to 60 mg. daily. Then adjusted to suit your needs.

Overdosage

Overdosage of prednisolone may result in anxiety; depression; confusion; high blood pressure; elevated blood sugar; stomach cramps or bleeding; swelling of the hands or feet; purplish skin patches. If you experience any of these symptoms, contact your doctor immediately, or go to a hospital emergency room. ALWAYS bring the medicine bottle with you.

Generic Name
Prednisone

Brand Names

Cortan
Deltasone
Fernisone
Meticorten
Orasone
Panasol
Prednicen-M
Sterapred
(Also available in generic form)

Type of Drug

Corticosteroid

Prescribed for

Rheumatoid arthritis; osteoarthritis; ankylosing spondylitis; acute gout; juvenile rheumatoid arthritis; psoriasis; systemic lupus erythematosus; polymyositis; many other nonarthritic conditions.

Cautions and Warnings

Avoid abrupt withdrawal of prednisone. Notify your doctor if, after having your dosage reduced or stopped, you experience fatigue; loss of appetite; weight loss; nausea; vomiting; diarrhea; weakness; dizziness.

Take prednisone with food to avoid upset stomach. Single daily doses, or every-other-day doses, should be taken preferably before 9:00 A.M. Multiple doses should be spread out evenly throughout the day.

Notify your doctor if you experience unusual weight gain; swelling of the ankles or feet; weakness; black tarry stools; vomiting of blood; heartburn; facial puffiness; menstrual irregularities; prolonged sore throat; fever; cold; infection. (Since prednisone may mask symptoms of infection, it is very important that you report anything that you suspect may be an infection.)

If you are taking prednisone, you should not be vaccinated against infectious diseases.

Pregnant women, women of childbearing potential, and nursing mothers should use prednisone only when the potential benefits clearly outweigh the unknown potential hazards to the fetus. If you become pregnant while taking prednisone, please notify your doctor.

Very stressful situations (such as an accident) may require an increase in dosage.

If you are on long-term prednisone therapy, you should wear or carry identification describing your medication.

If you are sensitive to aspirin or tartrazine, you may be allergic to prednisone.

Use with caution if you suffer from high blood pressure or kidney, liver, thyroid, or heart disease.

Your doctor may prescribe a calcium supplement to help prevent osteoporosis.

Possible Side Effects

Upset stomach; water retention; heart failure; potassium loss; muscle weakness; loss of muscle mass; calcium loss (osteoporosis); slow healing from wounds; black and blue marks; sweating; itching; rash; dizziness; headache.

Possible Adverse Effects

Slowing down of growth in children; depression of the adrenal and/or pituitary glands; diabetes; glaucoma; hypersensitivity or allergic reactions; blood clots; insomnia; weight gain; increased appetite; nausea; feeling of ill health. Psychic derangements may appear, ranging from euphoria to mood swings, personality changes, insomnia, and severe depression.

Drug Interactions

If you are diabetic, prednisone may cause the need for an increase in your antidiabetic medication.

Phenytoin, phenobarbital, rifampin, and possibly ephedrine may cause the need for an alteration in your prednisone dosage.

Prednisone may affect anticoagulant dosages.

Drugs that reduce serum-cholesterol levels, such as cholestyramine and colestipol, may decrease the effects of prednisone.

Interaction with diuretics may cause you to lose potassium. Be aware of signs of lowered potassium levels, such as weakness, muscle cramps, and tiredness, and report them to your doctor. Your doctor may recommend that you take a potassium supplement, or that you eat foods rich in potassium, such as bananas, citrus fruits, melon, and tomatoes.

Use aspirin with caution while taking prednisone.

Usual Dose

Initial dose: 5 to 60 mg. daily. Then adjusted to suit your needs.

Overdosage

Overdosage of prednisone may result in anxiety; depression; confusion; high blood pressure; elevated blood sugar; stomach cramps or bleeding; swelling of the hands or feet; purplish skin patches. If you experience any of these symptoms, contact your doctor immediately, or go to a hospital emergency room. ALWAYS bring the medicine bottle with you.

Generic Name
Probenecid

Brand Names

Benemid
Probalan
(Also available in generic form)

Type of Drug

Promotes the excretion of uric acid

Prescribed for

Gouty arthritis.

Cautions and Warnings

Avoid taking aspirin and other salicylates while taking probenecid.

Drink plenty of water (10 glasses per day) to prevent kidney-stone formation. Take probenecid with food to prevent upset stomach. Stomach problems may be the result of too high a dosage; therefore, notify your doctor if you suffer persistent upset stomach.

Probenecid may *worsen* gout attacks; in this case, treatment with colchicine is preferred.

Diabetics should note that probenecid may cause inaccurate results with copper sulfate urine sugar tests (Clinitest), but will give accurate results with a specific glucose enzymatic urine sugar test (Clinistix).

Pregnant women should use probenecid only when the benefits clearly outweigh the unknown potential hazards to the fetus.

Probenecid should not be taken by anyone who has a sensitivity to it, or by children under the age of 2.

Use probenecid with caution if you have a history of peptic ulcer, acute intermittent porphyria, and G-6-PD deficiency.

Your dosage of probenecid may have to be increased if you suffer from impaired kidney function.

Possible Side Effects

Headache; nausea; vomiting; loss of appetite; frequent urination; allergic skin reactions; flushing; dizziness.

Possible Adverse Effects

Sore gums, anemia. On rare occasions, kidney, liver, or blood diseases occur.

Drug Interactions

Do not take salicylates (i.e., aspirin) while taking probenecid.

Pyrazinamide interferes with the effect of probenecid.

Use methotrexate, sulfonamides, sulfonylureas, naproxen, indomethacin, rifampin, aminosalicylic acid, dapsone, clofibrate, and pantothenic acid with great caution when taking probenecid.

Usual Dose

0.25 gram twice a day for 1 week, followed by 0.5 gram twice daily.

If you suffer from a kidney impairment, a daily dose of 1 gram may be adequate. If necessary, this may be increased by 0.5-gram increments every 4 weeks, to 2 grams daily.

Overdose

There is no information available regarding probenecid overdose. However, if you think you are experiencing an overdose reaction, contact your doctor immediately, or go to a hospital emergency room. ALWAYS bring the medicine bottle with you.

Generic Name
Sulfinpyrazone

Brand Name

Anturane

Type of Drug

Promotes the excretion of uric acid

Prescribed for

Gouty arthritis.

Cautions and Warnings

Avoid aspirin and other salicylates while taking sulfinpyrazone.

Drink at least 10 to 12 glasses of water per day. Take sulfinpyrazone with food to prevent stomach upset.

Large doses of vitamin C may increase the possibility of forming kidney stones.

Do not take sulfinpyrazone if you suffer from an active peptic ulcer, gastrointestinal inflammation or ulceration, abnormal blood cells, or if you are allergic to phenylbutazone.

Pregnant women should use this drug only when the potential benefits clearly outweigh the unknown potential hazards to the fetus.

It is very important that you see your doctor on a regular basis while taking sulfinpyrazone. Periodic blood counts are recommended for patients undergoing long-term sulfinpyrazone treatment.

Possible Side Effects

Upset stomach; rash; bronchoconstriction.

Possible Adverse Effects

Abnormal blood cells; aggravation of peptic ulcer; reversible kidney dysfunction.

Drug Interactions

Salicylates (i.e., aspirin) should not be taken, because they decrease the effectiveness of sulfinpyrazone.

Sulfinpyrazone may increase the effects of coumarin-type anticoagulants (blood thinners), which may result in the need to adjust your anticoagulant dosage.

Use sulfinpyrazone with caution when taken with insulin, sulfa drugs, and oral antidiabetic drugs.

Usual Dose

Initial dose: 200 to 400 mg. daily in 2 divided doses.

Maintenance dose: 200 to 800 mg. daily.

Overdosage

Symptoms of an overdose reaction may include: nausea; vomiting; stomach pain; difficult breathing; lack of muscle control; convulsions; coma. If you think you are experiencing an overdose reaction, contact your doctor immediately, or go to a hospital emergency room. ALWAYS bring the medicine bottle with you.

Generic Name
Sulindac

Brand Name

Clinoril

Type of Drug

Nonsteroidal anti-inflammatory

Prescribed for

Rheumatoid arthritis, osteoarthritis, ankylosing spondylitis, acute gout, bursitis, tendinitis.

Cautions and Warnings

Do not use sulindac if you have had an allergic reaction to aspirin or any other nonsteroidal anti-inflammatory drug (NSAID).

Use with caution if you have a history of kidney, liver, or heart disease; high blood pressure; defects in the blood's clotting ability; or are currently taking anticoagulant medication. If you are suffering from an active peptic ulcer, it is recommended that other forms of drug therapy be tried before using sulindac.

With elderly patients, it is recommended that reduced dosages be instituted initially.

Use by pregnant women or nursing mothers is not recommended.

Anemia may occur in patients undergoing long-term therapy with sulindac. If you are anemic, it is suggested that you have your hemoglobin values determined frequently.

Pay special attention to any changes in your vision (blurred or partially obstructed vision or color blindness) or any eye complaints that occur when taking sulindac. Blurred vision is especially significant and requires a thorough eye examination. It is also recommended that you have your eyes checked regularly if you are undergoing prolonged therapy with sulindac.

Avoid aspirin while taking sulindac.

Sulindac may cause dizziness, drowsiness, or blurred vision; therefore, use caution while driving or performing tasks that require concentration.

To minimize upset stomach, take sulindac with food.

Possible Side Effects

Nausea; vomiting; diarrhea; constipation; upset stomach; dizziness; headache; drowsiness; nervousness; insomnia; asthma; heartburn; anemia.

Possible Adverse Effects

Irregular heartbeat; low blood pressure; chest pain; swelling of the hands or feet; adverse effects on the blood; unusual bleeding.

Drug Interactions

Using sulindac while taking anticoagulants may require a reduction of anticoagulant medication.

Aspirin may decrease the effectiveness of sulindac and probably should not be combined.

Probenecid may enhance the effects of sulindac; therefore, a reduced sulindac dosage may be necessary when taking probenecid.

Sulindac may increase the effects of anticonvulsants, antidiabetics, and sulfa drugs; your doctor may change the dosages of these other drugs.

Avoid alcohol, since this may increase stomach irritation and drowsiness.

Usual Dose

Rheumatoid arthritis, osteoarthritis, ankylosing spondylitis: Initial dose 150 mg. twice daily. Dosage is then adjusted to provide maximum benefits.

Bursitis, tendinitis, or *acute gout:* 200 mg. twice daily until pain subsides. Dosage is then reduced.

Safety and effectiveness for use by children has not been established.

Overdosage

In general, NSAID overdosage is treated by inducing vomiting, followed by the administration of activated charcoal. *However, do NOT induce vomiting or use activated charcoal unless directed to do so by your doctor or poison-control center.* When in doubt, proceed to a hospital emergency room. ALWAYS bring the medicine bottle with you.

Generic Name
Tolmetin Sodium

Brand Name

Tolectin

Type of Drug

Nonsteroidal anti-inflammatory

Prescribed for

Rheumatoid arthritis, juvenile rheumatoid arthritis, osteoarthritis.

Cautions and Warnings

Do not use tolmetin sodium if you have had an allergic reaction to aspirin or any other nonsteroidal anti-inflammatory drug (NSAID).

Use with caution if you have a history of kidney, liver, or heart disease; high blood pressure; defects in the blood's clotting ability; or are currently taking anticoagulant medication. If you are suffering from an active peptic ulcer, it is recommended that other forms of drug therapy be tried before using tolmetin sodium.

With elderly patients, it is recommended that reduced dosages be instituted initially.

Use by pregnant women or nursing mothers is not recommended.

Anemia may occur in patients undergoing long-term therapy with tolmetin sodium. If you are anemic, it is suggested that you have your hemoglobin values determined frequently.

Pay special attention to any changes in your vision (blurred or partially obstructed vision or color blindness) or any eye complaints that occur when taking tolmetin sodium. Blurred vision is especially significant and requires a thorough eye examination. It is also recommended that you have your eyes checked regularly if you are undergoing prolonged therapy with tolmetin sodium.

Avoid aspirin while taking tolmetin sodium.

Tolmetin sodium may cause dizziness, drowsiness, or blurred vision; therefore, use caution while driving or performing tasks that require concentration.

To minimize upset stomach, take tolmetin sodium with food.

Possible Side Effects

Nausea; vomiting; diarrhea; constipation; upset stomach; dizziness; headache; drowsiness; nervousness; insomnia; asthma; heartburn; anemia.

Possible Adverse Effects

Irregular heartbeat; low blood pressure; chest pain; swelling of the hands or feet; adverse effects on the blood; unusual bleeding.

Drug Interactions

Using tolmetin sodium while taking anticoagulants may require a reduction of anticoagulant medication.

Aspirin may decrease the effectiveness of tolmetin sodium and probably should not be combined.

Probenecid may enhance the effects of tolmetin sodium; therefore, a reduced tolmetin sodium dosage may be necessary when taking probenecid.

Tolmetin sodium may increase the effects of anticonvulsants, antidiabetics, and sulfa drugs; your doctor may change the dosages of these other drugs.

Avoid alcohol, since this may increase stomach irritation and drowsiness.

Do not take sodium bicarbonate with tolmetin sodium.

Usual Dose

Adults—rheumatoid arthritis and osteoarthritis: Initially 400 mg. 3 times daily. For rheumatoid arthritis the usual dosage is 600 to 1,800 mg. daily in divided doses. For osteoarthritis the usual dosage is 600 to 1,600 mg. daily in divided doses.

Children (2 years and older): Initially 9 mg. daily for every pound of body weight (given 3 or 4 times in divided doses). Do not give children more than 13.5 mg. daily per pound of body weight.

Overdosage

In general, NSAID overdosage is treated by inducing vomiting, followed by the administration of activated charcoal. *However, do NOT induce vomiting or use activated charcoal unless directed to do so by your doctor or poison-control center.* When in doubt, proceed to a hospital emergency room. ALWAYS bring the medicine bottle with you.

Generic Name

Triamcinolone

Brand Names

Aristocort
Kenacort
(Also available in generic form)

Type of Drug

Corticosteroid

Prescribed for

Rheumatoid arthritis; osteoarthritis; ankylosing spondylitis; acute gout; juvenile rheumatoid arthritis; psoriasis; systemic lupus erythematosus; polymyositis; many other nonarthritic conditions.

Cautions and Warnings

Avoid abrupt withdrawal of triamcinolone. Notify your doctor if, after having your dosage reduced or stopped, you experience fatigue; loss of appetite; weight loss; nausea; vomiting; diarrhea; weakness; dizziness.

Take triamcinolone with food to avoid upset stomach. Single daily doses, or every-other-day doses, should be taken preferably before 9:00 A.M. Multiple doses should be spread out evenly throughout the day.

Notify your doctor if you experience unusual weight gain; swelling of the ankles or feet; weakness; black tarry stools; vomiting of blood; heartburn; facial puffiness; menstrual irregularities; prolonged sore throat; fever; cold; infection. (Since triamcinolone may mask symptoms of infection, it is very important that you report anything that you suspect may be an infection.)

If you are taking triamcinolone, you should not be vaccinated against infectious diseases.

Pregnant women, women of childbearing potential, and nursing mothers should use triamcinolone only when the potential benefits clearly outweigh the unknown potential hazards to the fetus. If you become pregnant while taking triamcinolone, please notify your doctor.

Very stressful situations (such as an accident) may require an increase in dosage.

If you are on long-term triamcinolone therapy, you should wear or carry identification describing your medication.

If you are sensitive to aspirin or tartrazine, you may be allergic to triamcinolone.

Use with caution if you suffer from high blood pressure or kidney, liver, thyroid, or heart disease.

Your doctor may prescribe a calcium supplement to help prevent osteoporosis.

Possible Side Effects

Upset stomach; water retention; heart failure; potassium loss; muscle weakness; loss of muscle mass; calcium loss (osteoporosis); slow healing from wounds; black and blue marks; sweating; itching; rash; dizziness; headache.

Possible Adverse Effects

Slowing down of growth in children; depression of the adrenal and/or pituitary glands; diabetes; glaucoma; hypersensitivity or allergic reactions; blood clots; insomnia; weight gain; increased appetite; nausea; feeling of ill health. Psychic derangements may appear, ranging from euphoria to mood swings, personality changes, insomnia, and severe depression.

Drug Interactions

If you are diabetic, triamcinolone may cause the need for an increase in your antidiabetic medication.

Phenytoin, phenobarbital, rifampin, and possibly ephedrine may cause the need for an alteration in your triamcinolone dosage.

Triamcinolone may affect anticoagulant dosages.

Drugs that reduce serum-cholesterol levels, such as cholestyramine and colestipol, may decrease the effects of triamcinolone.

Interaction with diuretics may cause you to lose potassium. Be aware of signs of lowered potassium levels, such as weakness, muscle cramps, and tiredness, and report them to your doctor. Your doctor may recommend that you take a potassium supplement, or that you eat foods rich in potassium, such as bananas, citrus fruits, melon, and tomatoes.

Use aspirin with caution while taking triamcinolone.

Usual Dose

Rheumatic and dermatological disorders: Initial dose: 8 to 16 mg. daily. Then adjusted to suit your needs.

Systemic lupus erythematosus: Initial dose: 20 to 32 mg. daily. Then adjusted to suit your needs.

Overdosage

Overdosage of triamcinolone may result in anxiety; depression; confusion; high blood pressure; elevated blood sugar; stomach cramps or bleeding;

swelling of the hands or feet; purplish skin patches. If you experience any of these symptoms, contact your doctor immediately, or go to a hospital emergency room. ALWAYS bring the medicine bottle with you.

SOURCES

"Arthritis Experts Offer Advice to Hone Dx and Rx Skills." *Modern Medicine,* September 1981.

Berger, Bernard W., M.D., Ole J. Clemmensen, M.D., and A. Bernard Ackerman, M.D. "Lyme Disease Is a Spriochetosis." *The American Journal of Dermatopathology* 5, no. 2 (April 1983).

Boyd, J.R., ed. *Facts and Comparisons.* Philadelphia: J.B. Lippincott, 1984.

Brody, Jane E. "Arthritis: The Most Common Crippler." *The New York Times,* 14 October 1981.

Christensen, Jean. "Gout: Crystal Clear Diagnosis." *Aches & Pains,* October 1980.

Clark, Matt. "Here's Lead in Your Wine." *Newsweek,* 28 March 1983.

Copsey, Diana. "Steroid Joint Injections, Making Them More Effective." *Aches & Pains,* November 1980.

Delmar, Diana. "Measuring Patient Outcome in Arthritis." *Aches & Pains,* February 1981.

"Do's and Don't's in Arthritis," *Arthritis The Basic Facts,* The Arthritis Foundation, 1976.

Falk, Doris. "Shrinking Chronic Pain: How the Psychiatrist Can Work With You." *Aches & Pains,* November 1981.

———. "Juvenile Arthritis: Not Just in Children." *Aches & Pains,* April 1982.

Feder, Barnaby J. "The Boom in Arthritis Drugs." *The New York Times,* 23 April 1982.

"Filtering Rheumatoid Out of the Blood." *Science News,* 6 June 1981.

Fries, James F. *Arthritis: A Comprehensive Guide.* Reading, Mass.: Addison-Wesley, 1979.

Gall, Eric P., M.D. "The Safety of Treating Rheumatoid Arthritis With Aspirin." *Journal of the American Medical Association* 247, no. 1 (1 January 1982).

Goodwin, James S., M.D., Jan L. Ceuppens, M.D., and Martin A. Rodriguez, M.D. "Administration of Non-steroidal Anti-inflammatory Agents in Patients With Rheumatoid Arthritis." *British Medical Journal* 285 (4 December 1982).

Health Facts, Arthritis 6, no. 28 (July/August 1981). Center for Medical Consumers & Health Care Information, Inc.

"In Benoxaprofen's Wake, FDA Eyeing Drug Press Kits." *Medical World News,* 1 September 1982.

Katz, Warren A., M.D. *Rheumatic Diseases, Diagnosis and Management.* Philadelphia: J.B. Lippincott 1977.

The MacNeil-Lehrer Report. "Oraflex Controversy." New York: Educational Broadcasting Corporation and GWETA, 1982.

Marwick, Charles. "All Those Arthritis Drugs, How Do You Choose?" *Medical World News,* 2 August 1982.

Mayer, Jean, M.D. "No Form of Arthritis Can Be Eased By Diet." *Daily News,* 22 March 1974.

M.B. "The Pain of Arthritis." *Venture,* January 1983.

McCarty, Daniel, ed. *Arthritis & Allied Conditions,* Philadelphia: Lea & Febiger 1979.

"The Mistreatment of Arthritis." *Consumer Reports,* June 1979.

Neyens, Harry. "Sex and Arthritis." *Aches & Pains,* May 1981.

Physicians' Desk Reference, 38th ed. Oradell, N.J.: Medical Economics Company, 1984.

Pullar, T., H. A. Capell, A. Miller, and R. G. Brooks. "Alternative Medicine: Cost and Subjective Benefit in Rheumatoid Arthritis." *British Medical Journal* 285 (4 December 1982).

"Quackery in Arthritis Is Big Business." *The Arthritis Report.*

Roth, Sanford H. "The New Arthritis Drugs: How Much, How Often, How Long?" *Modern Medicine,* January 1983.

Scott, J. T. *Arthritis and Rheumatism: The Facts.* Oxford: Oxford University Press, 1980.

Willkens, Robert F., M.D. "The Use of Nonsteroidal Anti-inflammatory Agents." *Journal of the American Medical Association* 240, no. 15 (6 October 1978).

Winter, Ruth. "Arthritis Update." *Ladies Home Journal,* March 1977.

INDEX OF GENERIC AND BRAND NAME DRUGS

Generic drugs are printed in **boldface** type.

ABOUT THE MEDICAL CONSULTANT

Israeli A. Jaffe, M.D. is Professor of Clinical Medicine at the College of Physicians and Surgeons at Columbia University. He is currently attending physician at The Presbyterian Hospital in New York City. Dr. Jaffe, a world-reknowned medical researcher in the field of rheumatology, was director of the rheumatic disease program at the New York Medical College and associate director of a similar program at the Hospital for Joint Diseases-Orthopaedic Institute in New York City. Dr. Jaffe is a Fellow of the American College of Physicians and a certified Board Specialist by The American Board of Internal Medicine with a subspecialty in Rheumatology.

Dr. Jaffe is a graduate of the College of Physicians and Surgeons at Columbia University and was a clinical associate at the National Institute of Neurological Diseases and National Heart Institute. Dr. Jaffe was responsible for the discovery of the use of the drug Penicillamine in the treatment of severe rheumatoid arthritis. He is the author of over forty scientific and medical papers and reports. He has authored chapters in all of the standard arthritis textbooks. Dr. Jaffe lives with his wife and three children in New York City.

SPECIAL
MONEY SAVING
OFFER

Now you can have an up-to-date listing of Bantam's hundreds of titles plus take advantage of our unique and exciting bonus book offer. A special offer which gives you the opportunity to purchase a Bantam book for only 50¢. Here's how!

By ordering any five books at the regular price per order, you can also choose any other single book listed (up to a $4.95 value) for just 50¢. Some restrictions do apply, but for further details why not send for Bantam's listing of titles today!

Just send us your name and address plus 50¢ to defray the postage and handling costs.

How's Your Health?

Bantam publishes a line of informative books, written by top experts to help you toward a healthier and happier life.

NEED MORE INFORMATION ON YOUR HEALTH AND NUTRITION?

Read the books that will lead you to
a happier and healthier life.

We Deliver!
And So Do These Bestsellers.